# ISGE Series

**Series Editor**

Andrea R. Genazzani, Endocrinology, International Society of Gynecological Endocrinology, Pisa, Italy

The ISGE Book Series is the expression of the partnership between the International Society of Gynecological Endocrinology and Springer. The book series includes single monographs devoted to gynecological endocrinology relevant topics as well as the contents stemming from educational activities run by ISGRE, the educational branch of the society. This series is meant to be an important tool for physicians who want to advance their understanding of gynecological endocrinology and master this difficult clinical area. The International Society of Gynecological ad Reproductive Endocrinology (ISGRE) School fosters education and clinical application of modern gynecological endocrinology throughout the world by organizing high-level, highly focused residential courses twice a year, the Winter and the Summer Schools. World renowned experts are invited to provide their clinical experience and their scientific update to the scholars, creating a unique environment where science and clinical applications melt to provide the definitive update in this continuously evolving field. Key review papers are published in the Series, thus providing a broad overview over time on the major areas of gynecological endocrinology.

More information about this series at http://www.springer.com/series/11871

Andrea R. Genazzani • Michelle Nisolle •
Felice Petraglia • Robert N. Taylor
Editors

# Endometriosis Pathogenesis, Clinical Impact and Management

Volume 9: Frontiers in Gynecological Endocrinology

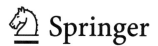

Springer

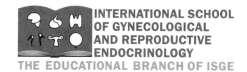

INTERNATIONAL SCHOOL
OF GYNECOLOGICAL
AND REPRODUCTIVE
ENDOCRINOLOGY
THE EDUCATIONAL BRANCH OF ISGE

*Editors*
Andrea R. Genazzani
International Society of Gynecological
Endocrinology
Pisa, Italy

Michelle Nisolle
Centre hospitalier régional de la Citad
Liège, Belgium

Felice Petraglia
Obstetrics and Gynecology Division
University of Florence
Firenze, Italy

Robert N. Taylor
Obstetrics & Gynecology Research Network
University of Utah
Salt Lake City, UT, USA

ISSN 2197-8735          ISSN 2197-8743   (electronic)
ISGE Series
ISBN 978-3-030-57868-8     ISBN 978-3-030-57866-4   (eBook)
https://doi.org/10.1007/978-3-030-57866-4

This Springer imprint is published by the registered company Springer Nature Switzerland AG.
The registered company address is: Gewerbestrasse 11, 6330 Cham, Switzerland

# Preface

Endometriosis is one of the most intriguing diseases for women during the reproductive age. It was almost a century ago (1921) that the first paper by John Sampson described the chocolate cysts of the ovary, and a few years later (1927), the publication which relates endometriosis to a "menstrual dissemination" came out. Anyhow, still today pathogenesis, diagnosis, and treatments of endometriosis are discussed.

The present book collects the most updated topics on endometriosis, and these will contribute to improve the knowledge of the disease and as consequence the management of the patients. The risk factors for women to develop endometriosis are a large variety, going from genetics to lifestyles, including the role of endocrine disruptor substances deriving from the environment (food, air). Starting from the concept that endometriosis is an endocrine/inflammatory disorder, the pathogenetic aspects of endometriosis are discussed in terms of immunological factors and metabolomic characteristics. The clinical implication of this basic science study is to discover new tools for a noninvasive diagnosis of endometriosis, considering that imaging is already offering good parameters for an early diagnosis of endometriosis.

Pain and infertility are the major symptoms of women with endometriosis and both highly reduce their quality of life. The incidence of endometriosis in adolescent girls is increasing and the debate is open in terms of diagnosis and treatments (progestins, combined oral contraceptive, or surgery) and in the long-term management. The ovarian endometriosis, endometrioma, is the most common phenotype and evidences are suggesting to be very cautious and conservative in the surgical treatment because it affects ovarian reserve. In the case that patients with endometriosis desire a pregnancy, infertility is an important issue, and the role of surgery in order to improve pregnancy outcome is discussed, in comparison with ART technologies and embryo characteristics. The correlation of endometriosis with ovarian cancer and menopausal symptoms are topics under discussion.

The present book aims to offer to the gynecologists a modern and updated picture of endometriosis. The molecular and clinical characteristics of the disease are changing in the new millennium and an update on basic and clinical aspects of endometriosis is relevant for helping clinicians to approach a modern management of these patients.

Pisa, Italy                                              Andrea R. Genazzani
Liege, Belgium                                            Michelle Nisolle
Firenze, Italy                                            Felice Petraglia
Salt Lake City, UT, USA                                    Robert Taylor

# Contents

# Endocrine Disruptors and Endometriosis Risk

Marco Palumbo and Federica Di Guardo

## 1.1 Introduction

Endometriosis is defined as the presence of endometrial-type mucosa outside the uterine cavity. Several theories have been proposed during the last 20 years to explain the disease pathogenesis; however, a unique consensus has not yet been established. Although the most recent pathogenic theory is based on inflammatory causes [1], hormonal influence is certainly involved not only in the endometriosis pathogenesis but also in its development and progression [2].

Ectopic endometrium seems, in fact, to be dependent on estrogens and to be resistant to progesterone. Estradiol, which represents the active form of estrogens, is hyper expressed in endometriosis tissue and acts as a transcription factor due to the capacity to link to nuclear receptors. In the same way, chemical environment substances can act as binding endogenous hormone receptors and are therefore called "endocrine disruptors." These chemical compounds are able to bind the estrogen and progesterone receptor, as well as determining pro-inflammatory effects, and in this context, they may be potential risk factors for the development of endometriosis.

## 1.2 Endocrine Disruptors

In 2012, the United Nations Environment Programme (UNEP) and the World Health Organization (WHO) prepared a report entitled "State of Science: Endocrine Distrupting Chemicals-2012." This document described about 800 chemicals

M. Palumbo (✉) · F. Di Guardo
Department of General Surgery and Medical-Surgical Specialties, University of Catania, Catania, Italy
e-mail: marcoànt.palumbo@tiscali.it

© International Society of Gynecological Endocrinology 2021
A. R. Genazzani et al. (eds.), *Endometriosis Pathogenesis, Clinical Impact and Management*, ISGE Series, https://doi.org/10.1007/978-3-030-57866-4_1

**Table 1.1** Endocrine disruptors interacting with female endocrine system receptors

| Chemical compounds | Pathways of exposures | Hormonal activity |
|---|---|---|
| DDT and metabolites | Milk and derivatives, fatty fish, living environment and workplaces | Estrogenic activity |
| Organochlorine insecticides | Milk and derivatives, fatty fish, living environment, workplaces | Interaction with progesterone receptors, estrogenic and/or anti-androgenic activity |
| Nonyl-phenols and octyl-phenols | Detergent by-products: Food chain (seafood) and consumer products | Estrogen agonists—ER α |
| Bisphenol A | Detergent by-products: Food chain (seafood) and consumer products | Estrogen agonist—ER α |
| Several phthalates (di-2-hexyl-ethyl-, di-$n$-butyl-, etc.) | Plastics in contact with food, consumer products (e.g., PVC, deodorants, adhesives, etc.) | Estrogen agonists—ER α |
| Parabens | Cosmetic products | Estrogen agonist—ER α and β |
| UV-screen (benzophenone 2, 4-methylbenzylidene camphor, etc.) | Mixture for protection against UV radiation | Estrogen agonist—ER α |
| Cadmium | Flour, rice, sugar, seafood, cigarette smoking | Estrogen agonist—ER α |
| Isoflavones, lignans, etc. | Vegetables, soy-based food, cosmetics | SERMs, high affinity for ER β |

suspected of being endocrine disrupters able of mimicking endogenous hormones or altering their regulation [3].

An endocrine disrupter is defined as an exogenous substance or mixture that can disturb the functions of the endocrine system and cause adverse health effects in the body or in the population [4].

Endocrine disruptors may act altering the production, secretion, metabolism, transport, or peripheral action of endogenous hormones binding to hormone receptors.

After binding the receptors, the results can manifest as an agonistic effect (mimicking the hormonal action) or antagonistic effect (contrasting the hormonal action by preventing the binding of the natural hormone). Endocrine disruptors may also be capable of binding allosteric sites, producing unexpected effects at very low concentrations.

In addition, these substances can also act by recruiting co-activators or co-expressers in various enzymatic pathways, modifying hormone synthesis, plasma clearance, or gene expression through epigenetic alterations.

Considering the response curve of these compounds, their adverse effects are not directly proportional to the exposure dose, meaning that very low quantity also could have significant effects on cell proliferation and development, creating problems for the human risk assessment [5].

Endocrine disrupters include a large and variegate group in terms of use, chemical structure, and mode of action (Table 1.1). Among them, there are persistent pollutants capable of bio-accumulation (dioxins, DDT, and cadmium), chemical substances used in plant or animal feed production (azole fungicides, etc.). Bisphenol A (BPA) and Di-(2-ethylhexyl) phthalate (DEHP) deserve a special mention, in order of their wide use in industry or consumer products (plastic bottles and other daily-life products) causing, therefore, continued exposure to humans. Phytoestrogens (hormonally active compounds of plant origin) are also included in the endocrine disrupters category.

As hormones may act on distant site target organs, in the same way the endocrine disruptors are supposed to affect several hormone pathways, making it difficult to understand their full mechanism of action [6].

However, the effects tend to be tissue-specific, in order of the fact that chemical substances are metabolized in specific sites. Resulting metabolites seem to interfere with hormone actions in the same tissues where they were generated. In addition, some tissues exhibit a higher receptor density or different receptor isoforms [7].

Endocrine disruptors have a broad spectrum of action on human health including effects on the development of reproductive and nervous systems, metabolism, and cancer.

They can act as determining indirect epigenetic molecular alterations at the germline level having a role in determining effects on subsequent generations. This phenomenon is called "trans-generational inheritance" [8, 9].

Moreover, several epidemiological studies have linked the direct individual exposure to endocrine disruptors with effects on the female endocrine system and reproductive tract (Table 1.1): early puberty, aneuploidy, polycystic ovary syndrome, early ovarian failure, and menstrual and fertility changes [8, 10].

### 1.2.1 Focus on BPA and Phthalates

Bisphenol A (BPA) is an industrial chemical substance found in synthetic plastics: it is the main intermediate in the synthesis of polycarbonate polymers and epoxy resins, as well as a component of some polyvinyl chloride plastic. These materials are widely used in products such as feeding bottles, coating of food, beverage containers, and dental fillings. Human exposure to BPA migrates from plastic products to food or water during the heating process, capable of breaking the external bonds that allow the substance to be a polymer. This results in direct exposure to humans [11].

Phthalates are also widely used in consumer products, including food packaging, medical devices, and toys, mainly to improve the flexibility and durability of polyvinyl chloride plastics. Phthalates are not covalently bound to the plastic matrix, and therefore, they can be easily released into the environment. Recent epidemiological evidences suggest that women have an increased exposure to phthalates compared to men, as they are present in beauty products, including skin lotions, perfumes, and nail products. In particular, di-(2-ethylhexyl) phthalate (DEHP) represents the most used compound [12].

According to the lines above, the main route of exposure to the aforementioned compound is the oral route, followed by the inhalation and the dermal route [11].

BPA and phthalates are rapidly metabolized and excreted in urine without evidence of accumulation in the body; the elimination is considered complete within 24 h of exposure [13].

## 1.2.2 BPA and Phthalates Mechanisms of Action

The mechanism of action of BPA and phthalates is complex because they are not strictly specific in their binding to the hormone receptors.

BPA is a 2,2-bis(4-hydroxyphenyl)-propane, containing two functional phenolic groups that allow the substance to interact with the estrogen and androgen receptor, both as an agonist and as an antagonist [14].

Due to this interaction with the estrogen receptor (ER) α and ER β, the mechanism of action of the BPA is expressed through the ER-dependent signaling pathways. According to this, three well-characterized ER target genes were examined: GREB1 (estrogen regulation in breast cancer 1), PGR (progesterone receptor), and WISP-2/CNN5 (protein 2 of the WWT1-inducible signaling pathway). BPA has been shown to significantly induce these target genes mediating transcriptional activity via ER [15].

Bond assays for nuclear ER and transcriptional activation assays indicate that BPA has at least 10,000 times less affinity for the two nuclear estrogen receptors than Estradiol. This would suggest that BPA exposure is not significant if it occurs at environmental low levels. However, there is evidence that once tolerable exposure conditions have passed (below the threshold of 50 µg/kg body weight/day), BPA effects may be added to those of ovarian estrogens. According to some in vitro experiments, BPA can even act as Estradiol equivalent in some cellular endpoint systems. In accord with recent evidences acquired on the mimetic estrogens functioning in non-genomic signal pathways, BPA is capable of triggering signal cascades by binding to estrogens membrane receptors (in particular the GPR30 receptor). In this context, BPA behaves as SERM (selective modulators of the membrane estrogen receptor) capable of alternating with transcriptional co-modulators (histone acetyltransferase and histone deacetylase) to mediate different responses depending on the target tissue [16].

Other important BPA-related receptors are the aryl hydrocarbon receptors (AhR), peroxisome proliferator-activated receptors (PPAR), and Toll-like receptors (TLR) [17].

Phthalates are synthetic esters of phthalic anhydride. The chemical structure of each individual phthalate varies, mainly according to the expression of the lateral chains and molecular weight. They can be grouped into two broad categories: low-weight and high-weight phthalates.

Low molecular weight phthalates include dimethyl phthalate (DMP), diethyl phthalate (DEP), and dibutyl phthalate (DBP). High molecular weight phthalates include diethyl hexyl phthalate (DEHP), diisononyl phthalate (DINP), diisodecyl phthalate (DIDP), and benzyl butyl phthalate (BBzP) [18].

In contrast to BPA, phthalates do not appear to act by direct hormonal bounding; however, some of these including di(2-ethylhexyl) phthalate (DEHP) have been shown to have estrogenic activity in in vitro assays [19] as well as modulating androgen production. In this context, DEHP produces anti-androgenic effects through the reduction of testosterone production. It is also capable of binding and activating the receptors activated by the peroxisome proliferator (PPAR) [20] and the thyroid hormone receptor [9].

## 1.3 Endocrine Disruptors and Endometriosis: Literature Evidences

Endometriosis has been described as an estrogen-dependent pathology, in which onset and progression are involved alterations in endometrium steroidogenesis and peritoneal cavity balance, with excessive estrogen production from ectopic endometriosis lesions. It is therefore plausible that endocrine disruptors, who mimic or alter endogenous hormonal activity, may influence the risk of endometriosis and be involved in its development and progression.

In this scenario, positive associations have been found between persistent environmental exposure to organochlorine pesticides and endometriosis [21].

Several studies have also confirmed the role of the environmental contaminant 2,3,7,8-tetrachlorodibenzo-*p*-dioxin (TCDD), commonly known as dioxin, as a potential risk factor for the development of endometriosis [22, 23]. There is also a strong association between uterine exposure to diethylstilbestrol (DES) (prescribed from the 1940s to the 1970s for high-risk pregnancies to prevent miscarriage) and the development of endometriosis later in adult life, as well as other reproductive abnormalities such as cervical and vaginal hypoplasia, infertility, early menopause, and a rare case of clear-cell vaginal adenocarcinoma [24].

Considering the ability of BPA and phthalates to interact with ER, they may be involved in estrogen-dependent diseases such as endometriosis. In addition, BPA decreases PR progesterone receptor expression, as demonstrated by a primate model study in which PR expression decreased more after treatment with BPA and estradiol than after treatment with estradiol alone. In this way, the ability of progesterone to inhibit the action of estradiol on the endometrium is reduced, leading to increased endometrial proliferation [25]. Thus, BPA would also contribute to the "progesterone-resistance" phenomenon found in endometriosis.

On the other hand, recent studies have found pro-inflammatory responses induced by phthalates through the binding and activation of the receptor activated by the peroxisome proliferator (PPAR) and this can be related to endometriosis, a disease involving oxidative stress and inflammation [20]. Moreover, recent in vitro studies suggested that DEHP could increase the reactive oxygen species (ROS) generation and decrease the expression of superoxide dismutase (SOD). In this way, it seems to induce the ER α expression in a dose-dependent manner: the result can be the development of endocrine-related disease including endometriosis [26].

Laboratory tests have shown an endometriosis-like phenotype within the female offspring of mice exposed to BPA and phthalates in the perinatal phase [27].

This means that the disease has been induced by alterations during female embryological development through changes in genic and epigenetic modulation. This is in line with "embryonic theory" as a pathogenic hypothesis of endometriosis.

In contrast to laboratory studies, epidemiological studies have not given consistent results regarding the association between the levels of BPA and DEHP and endometriosis.

Literature evidences had shown a positive association between concentrations of the aforementioned substances in women with endometriosis and those without endometriosis [28–31].

A study conducted by Buck Louis [32] found a positive correlation between urinary levels of phthalate metabolites and diagnosis of endometriosis but found no such correlation with BPA. Even a cross-sectional Japanese study found no correlation between the urinary concentration of BPA and endometriosis compared to the daily expected concentration in the general population [33]. On the other hand, a case–control study of Upson showed an increase in urinary BPA levels in women with endometriosis compared to healthy women, but limited to cases of non-ovarian pelvic endometriosis; concentrations with ovarian endometriosis were not statistically significant [34]. Conversely, Rashidi found a positive correlation between higher BPA in the urine of women with ovarian endometriosis compared to healthy controls [35].

To the best of our knowledge, there is consistent evidence demonstrating that exposure to endocrine disruptors has a connection with the incidence of endometriosis.

Co-exposure to several endocrine disruptors (humans are most likely to be exposed to a mixture of chemicals rather than a single chemical) may exacerbate toxicological effects via different pathogenic mechanisms and targets tissues. Adequate sample size, occupational exposure, longitudinal investigation, and multi-center clinical studies need to be conducted trying to focus on pathogenic mechanism, on exposure dose, and exposure duration. Co-exposure to endocrine disruptors need to be further investigated in order to understand their interactions and make the existent evidence more credible.

## References

1. Sourial S, Tempest N, Hapangama DK. Theories on the pathogenesis of endometriosis. Int J Reprod Med. 2014;2014:179515.
2. Di Guardo F, et al. Management of women affected by endometriosis: are we stepping forward? J Endo Pelvic Pain Dis. 2019;11(2):77–84.
3. Roy D, et al. Integrated bioinformatics, environmental epidemiologic and genomic approaches to identify environmental and molecular links between endometriosis and breast Cancer. Int J Mol Sci. 2015;16(10):25285–322.
4. Preciados M, et al. Estrogenic endocrine disrupting chemicals influencing NRF1 regulated gene networks in the development of complex human brain disease. Int J Mol Sci. 2016;17(12):2086.

5. Welshons WV, et al. Large effects from small exposures. I. Mechanisms for endocrine-disrupting chemicals with estrogenic activity. Environ Health Perspect. 2003;111(8):994–1006.
6. Borgeest C, et al. The effects of endocrine disrupting chemicals on the ovary. Front Biosci. 2002;7:d1941–8.
7. Zoeller RT, et al. Endocrine-disrupting chemicals and public health protection: a statement of principles from the Endocrine Society. Endocrinology. 2012;153(9):4097–110.
8. Street ME, et al. Current knowledge on endocrine disrupting chemicals (EDCs) from animal biology to humans, from pregnancy to adulthood: highlights from a national Italian meeting. Int J Mol Sci. 2018;19(6):1647.
9. Skinner MK. Endocrine disruptors in 2015: epigenetic transgenerational inheritance. Nat Rev Endocrinol. 2016;12(2):68–70.
10. Craig ZR, et al. Endocrine-disrupting chemicals in ovarian function: effects on steroidogenesis, metabolism and nuclear receptor signaling. Reproduction. 2011;142(5):633–46.
11. Li X, Frank AA. Improvement of bisphenol A quantitation from urine by LCMS. Anal Bioanal Chem. 2015;407(13):3869–74.
12. Kim JH. Analysis of the in vitro effects of di-(2-ethylhexyl) phthalate exposure on human uterine leiomyoma cells. Exp Ther Med. 2018;15(6):4972–8.
13. Germaine M, et al. Bisphenol A and phthalates and endometriosis, the ENDO study. Fertil Steril. 2013;100(1):162–9.
14. Michalowicz J. Bisphenol A-sources toxicity and biotransformation. Environ Toxicol Pharmacol. 2014;37(2):738–58.
15. Li Y, et al. Differential in vitro biological action, coregulator interactions, and molecular dynamic analysis of bisphenol A (BPA), BPAF, and BPS ligand-ERa complexes. Environ Health Perspect. 2018;126(1):017012.
16. Watson CS, et al. Nongenomic signaling pathways of estrogen toxicity. Toxicol Sci. 2010;115(1):1–11.
17. Xu J, et al. Developmental Bisphenol A exposure modulates immune-related diseases. Toxics. 2016;4(4):23.
18. North ML, et al. Effects of phthalates on the development and expression of allergic disease and asthma. Ann Allergy Asthma Immunol. 2014;112(6):496–502.
19. Okubo T, et al. Estimation of estrogenic and anti-estrogenic activities of some phthalate diesters and monoesters by MCF-7 cell proliferation assay in vitro. Biol Pharm Bull. 2003;26:1219–24.
20. Ferguson KK, et al. Associations between maternal biomarkers of phthalate exposure and inflammation using repeated measurements across pregnancy. PLoS One. 2015;10(8):90135601.
21. Upson K, et al. Organochlorine pesticides and risk of endometriosis: findings from a population-based case-control study. Environ Health Perspect. 2013;121(11–12):1319–24.
22. Igarashi T, et al. Expression of Ah receptor and dioxin-related genes in human uterine endometrium in women with or without endometriosis. Endocr J. 1999;46:765–72.
23. Bruner-Tran KL, et al. Dioxin may promote inflammation-related development of endometriosis. Fertil Steril. 2008;89(5 Suppl):1287–98.
24. Missmer SA, et al. In utero exposures and the incidence of endometriosis. Fertil Steril. 2004;82(6):1501–8.
25. Aldad TS, et al. Bisphenol-A exposure alters endometrial progesterone receptor expression in the nonhuman primate. Fertil Steril. 2011;96(1):175–9.
26. Cho YJ, Park SB, Han M. Di-(2-ethylhexyl)-phthalate induces oxidative stress in human endometrial stromal cells in vitro. Mol Cell Endocrinol. 2015;407:9–17.
27. Signorile PG, et al. Pre-natal exposure of mice to bisphenol A elicits an endometriosis-like phenotype in female offspring. Gen Comp Endocrinol. 2010;168(3):318–25.
28. Cobellis L, et al. High plasma concentrations of di-(2-ethylhexyl)-phthalate in women with endometriosis. Hum Reprod. 2003;18(7):1512–5.
29. Kim SH, et al. Increased plasma levels of phthalate esters in women with advanced-stage endometriosis: a prospective case-control study. Fertil Steril. 2011;95(1):357–9.

30. Cobellis L, et al. Measurement of bisphenol A and bisphenol B levels in human blood sera from healthy and endometriotic women. Biomed Chromatogr. 2009;23(11):1186–9.
31. Weuve J, et al. Association of exposure to phthalates with endometriosis and uterine leiomyomata: findings from NHANES, 1999–2004. Environ Health Perspect. 2010;118 (6):825–3.
32. Louis B, et al. Bisphenol A and phthalates and endometriosis, the ENDO study. Fertil Steril. 2013;100(1):162–169.e2.
33. Itoh H, et al. Urinary bisphenol-A concentration in infertile Japanese women and its association with endometriosis: a cross-sectional study. Environ Health Prev Med. 2007;12:258–64.
34. Upson K, et al. A population-based case-control study of urinary bisphenol A concentration and risk of endometriosis. Hum Reprod. 2014;29(11):2457–64.
35. Rashidi BH. A case-control study of Bisphenol A and endometrioma among subgroup of Iranian women. J Res Med Sci. 2017;22:7.

# Metabolomic Characteristics in Endometriosis Patients

Stefano Angioni, Stefania Saponara, Antonio G. Succu, Marco Sigilli, Francesco Scicchitano, and Maurizio N. D'Alterio

## 2.1 Introduction

Endometriosis is an oestrogen-dependent disease, characterised by the presence of abnormal endometrial tissue (glands and stroma) outside the uterus, mainly localised within the pelvis (peritoneum, ovaries, recto-vaginal space, urinary tract) [1], as well as in extra-pelvic sites (lung, brain, umbilicus and surgical scars) [2]. Endometriosis is the most common benign gynaecological disease affecting women of reproductive age and is one of the most frequent causes of infertility [3]. Estimating the exact prevalence of endometriosis is still challenging, since many women with this pathology are asymptomatic and the diagnosis is often overlooked by many doctors; on average, its diagnosis is delayed for an average of 10 years [3]. The prevalence of the disease seems to be ~5%, with a peak between 25 and 35 years of age; it tends to regress after menopause [3]. Endometriosis can take one of these forms: peritoneal or superficial endometriosis, ovarian endometrioma (OMA), or deep infiltrating endometriosis (DIE) [4]. Common clinical manifestations of endometriosis are chronic pelvic pain, dysmenorrhoea, dyschezia/constipation and dysuria, depending on the affected site. The symptoms may have a significant negative impact on a patient's quality of life [5]. The diagnosis of endometriosis is difficult because of the prevalence of aspecific symptoms, its late presentation and the dependence on a physician's personal conviction and local diagnostic-therapeutic paths and expertise in order to make a diagnosis. The diagnosis is frequently performed by physical examination associated with transvaginal ultrasonography (TVUS), which is the first-line imaging technique, and magnetic resonance imaging (MRI) [6]. Laparoscopic visualisation has generally been considered the gold standard for endometriosis diagnosis [7]. However, the use of laparoscopy is limited by available funding, a surgeon's experience, and human error, including missing aspecific

S. Angioni (✉) · S. Saponara · A. G. Succu · M. Sigilli · F. Scicchitano · M. N. D'Alterio
Department of Surgical Sciences, University of Cagliari, Cagliari, Italy

© International Society of Gynecological Endocrinology 2021
A. R. Genazzani et al. (eds.), *Endometriosis Pathogenesis, Clinical Impact and Management*, ISGE Series, https://doi.org/10.1007/978-3-030-57866-4_2

lesions. Currently, physicians rely on clinical diagnosis to start medical treatment, while laparoscopy is still indicated only in specific cases [8]. In addition to instrumental diagnostics, historically, the only marker utilised in clinical practice and detectable in serum is CA125, which increases in endometriosis, especially in advanced cases [9]. Unfortunately, its levels are also increased in epithelial ovarian cancer and vary significantly during the menstrual cycle. In general, CA125 and other proposed markers have not shown promising outcomes in terms of diagnostic value [10]. Recently, research approaches have been focusing on new, non-invasive tools for the early diagnosis of endometriosis [11]. *Metabolomics* is a new field of study, belonging to the omic sciences, which focuses on small molecule metabolites with the aim of clarifying the pathogenesis of different diseases or identifying biomarkers that may be useful for their diagnosis.

## 2.2    Omics Sciences

The word *omics* refers to the collective technologies used to evaluate roles, relationships and actions of different molecules that compose the cells of an organism. These technologies include genomics (the study of genes and their function), proteomics (the study of proteins), transcriptomics (the study of mRNA) glycomics (the study of carbohydrates cellular) and lipomics (the study of cellular lipids) [12]. Metabolomics can be conceptually defined as 'the quantitative measure of the global and dynamic metabolic response of living systems to biological impulses or genetic modifications,' allowing for identification and quantification of the low molecular weight metabolites that can act as mediators of the pathological cellular responses [13]. Mass spectrometry (MS) and magnetic resonance imaging (MRI) are very useful for metabolomic study. Compared to MRI, MS has a higher sensitivity for detecting infinitesimal concentrations of a metabolite in biological samples [14]. On the other hand, MRI is highly reproducible, allows for quantitative analysis and does not require additional technical preparation steps, such as separation or derivation of the sample [14].

MRI and MS can both detect amino acids, nucleosides, nucleotides, sugars and organic acids in different samples like endometrial [15] and follicular fluid [16], urine [17], serum [18] and plasma [19] (Tables 2.1 and 2.2).

## 2.3    Metabolomic Approach in the Diagnosis of Endometriosis

As a response to catabolic damage, endometriosis is characterised by a higher protein turnover, which means that a higher level of metabolites (amino acids) are released into the bloodstream [20]. Considering that the endometrial tissue communicates directly and indirectly (through extracellular fluids) with blood circulation, some of these metabolites have been studied in patients' serum for the diagnosis of endometriosis. Dutta et al. demonstrated that endometrial tissue samples of patients with endometriosis had a lower level of alanine, lysine, phenylalanine and

**Table 2.1**  Principal biomarkers identified in serum in patients affected by endometriosis

| Biomarkers | Serum concentration | References |
|---|---|---|
| *Amino acids* | | |
| Alanine | ↑ | Dutta et al. [11] |
| Lysine | ↑ | Dutta et al. [18] |
| Phenylalanine | ↑ | |
| Leucine | ↑ | |
| Valine | ↑ | |
| Threonine | ↑ | |
| Taurine | ↑ | |
| Arginine | ↓ | |
| Isoleucine | ↓ | |
| *Lipids* | | |
| Sphyngomielins | ↑ | Vouk et al. [19] |
| Ether-phospholipids | ↑ | |
| *Sugars* | | |
| Glucose | ↓ | Dutta et al. [18] |
| *Organic acids* | | |
| Lactate | ↑ | Dutta et al. [18] |
| 2-Hydroxybutyrate | ↑ | |
| 3-Hydroxybutyrate | ↑ | |
| *Other metabolites* | | |
| 2-Methoxyestradiol | ↑ | Ghazi et al. [33] |
| 2-Methoxyestrone | ↑ | |
| Dehydroepiandrosterone | ↑ | |
| Androstenedione | ↑ | |
| Cholesterol | ↑ | |
| Acyl-carnitine (long-chain) | ↑ | Vouk et al. [19] |
| Primitive bile acids | ↓ | Ghazi et al. [33] |

leucine levels, whereas higher levels of these metabolites were found in serum samples [11]. They found that for the rASRM (revised American Society for Reproductive Medicine) stage I (minimal) diagnosis, alanine showed 90% sensitivity and 58% specificity. For Stage II (mild) diagnosis, Phenylalanine was revealed as the most sensible marker (100%), whereas its specificity is 75%. Leucine showed maximum specificity of 91.7%, while its sensitivity is set at 69.2%. Further, they generated a regression model with a panel of serum markers showing an improved sensitivity of 100% and specificity of 83%, for Stage II diagnosis [11].

Since endometriosis is considered a chronic inflammatory disease, with alterations of the immune system and high levels of cytokines and growth factors in peritoneal fluid, the study of energetic metabolism is mandatory [21]. Immune and inflammatory diseases are characterised by an abnormal amount of energy consumption, deriving from precursors like glucose, glutamine, ketone bodies and fatty acids [18–22]. Recent studies have shown altered glutamine and glutamate levels in endometrial tissue of patients affected endometriosis [11]. Glutamine is mainly produced in muscular tissue, as well as in the brain and lungs, even if in lower

**Table 2.2** Principal biomarkers id↑entified in other samples in patients affected by endometriosis

| Biomarkers | Sample | Concentration | References |
|---|---|---|---|
| *Amino acids* | | | |
| Alanine | Endometrial tissue | ↓ | Dutta et al. [11] |
| Lysine | Endometrial tissue | ↓ | |
| Phenylalanine | Endometrial tissue | ↓ | |
| Leucine | Endometrial tissue | ↓ | |
| Glutamine | Cerebral tissue | ↑ | As-Sanie et al. [22] |
| Taurine | Urine sample | ↑ | Vincente-Muñoz et al. [17] |
| Valine | Urine sample | ↑ | |
| *Lipids* | | | |
| Monohexosylceramides | Endometrial fluid | ↓ | Dominguez et al. [15] |
| Ceramides | Endometrial fluid | ↓↑ | |
| Glycerophospholipids | Endometrial fluid | ↑ | |
| Glycerolipids | Endometrial fluid | ↑ | |
| Phosphatidylcholines | Follicular fluid | ↑ | Cordeiro et al. [16] |
| *Other metabolites* | | | |
| Estradiol | Adipose and peripheral tissue | ↑ | Hashim et al. [31] |
| N1-Metil-4-pyridone-5 carboxamide | Urine sample | ↑ | Vincente-Muñoz et al. [17] |
| Guanidino-succinate | Urine sample | ↑ | |
| Creatinine | Urine sample | ↑ | |
| 2-Hydroxyisovalerate | Urine sample | ↑ | |
| Formate | Endometriotic tissue | ↓ | Dutta et al. [11] |

levels. Recently, As-Sanie et al. have shown high amounts of glutamine in the cerebral tissue of women affected by endometriosis, particularly in the insula region, supposing its involvement in chronic pelvic pain genesis and perception in these women [22]. These findings may represent a new opportunity to perform a non-invasive diagnosis of endometriosis and help us to differentiate between asymptomatic patients with endometriosis and patients who have chronic pelvic pain but do not have endometriosis.

It is widely accepted that endometriotic cells, similarly to neoplastic cells, have a great proliferative, implantation and neo-angiogenetic ability, thus having the possibility to adapt to the unfavourable conditions of an ectopic environment [23]. Some recent evidence has suggested that such properties could be already characteristic of eutopic endometrial cells before they migrate elsewhere in the body [24]. Focusing on the comparison between endometriotic and neoplastic cells, some authors have analysed different metabolites, like taurine and myo-inositol [25]. Taurine is a ß-amino acid detectable in high levels in neoplastic cells and associated with an increased proliferation rate. Myo-inositol is the active form of inositol (a sugar similar to glucose), and it is involved in different cellular signalling processes, and when associated with lipids, it has structural functions [25]. High levels of these two metabolites result in the tissue of advanced stages of endometriosis, thus presenting similarity to prostate cancer [26] and squamous cell carcinomas [27]. In moderate and severe endometriosis, endometriotic cells need to increase their nucleotides synthesis to continue the neoangiogenic process, depleting molecules like formate, which is incorporated in purine nucleotides; this may explain why low formate levels are found in endometriotic tissues in the advanced stages of the disease [11]. Another similarity between endometriosis and cancer is the pyruvate metabolism alteration with a consequent increase of lactates and a significative decrease of serum glucose level [18]. These modifications indicate an elevated anaerobic activity, even in the presence of adequate oxygen levels. This effect is also known as the *Warburg effect* [28]. Anaerobic glycolysis is also characterised by elevated levels of alanine, valine and 3-hydroxybutyrate. An increased serum concentration of these metabolites was also found in advanced stages of endometriosis [18] and some epithelial ovarian cancers [29]. In serum of patients with endometriosis, reduced glutathione (GSH) levels are also detected, as a result of high reactive oxygen species (ROS) process and high cellular oxidative stress. This GSH deficit results in increased ophthalmate synthesis, which generates 2-hydroxybutyrate, becoming another possible marker of cellular oxidative stress in patients with endometriosis [18].

Furthermore, as a reflex of energetic metabolism involvement, acyl-carnitine may represent a new marker of the disease [30]. This compound is composed of esterified fatty acids with a carnitine molecule and its role is to carry fatty acids through the inner mitochondrial membrane. Because endometriosis is characterised by a chronic inflammatory state, the excessive heat generation may affect the efficiency of mitochondrial enzymes involved in the beta-oxidation process [19]. Recent data support these findings by showing an increased plasma level of long-chain acyl-carnitines and higher long-chain/medium-chain acyl-carnitines rate [19].

Other authors have shown increased aromatase activity, which leads to a higher synthesis of oestradiol in adipose and peripheral tissues [31], whereas its serum levels remained unchanged [32]. Ghazi et al. found five metabolites that were significantly increased in the serum of women with endometriosis: 2-methoxyestradiol, 2-methoxyestrone, dehydroepiandrosterone, androstenedione and cholesterol [33]. By researching specific oestradiol metabolites in serum and urine, high levels of 2-methoxyestradiol, 2-methoxyestrone have been found [32]. Furthermore, Ghazi et al. showed also a significant reduction in serum bile acid metabolites, which are essential for liver oestrogen excretion; this decrease may lead to a hyper-oestrogenic state and, consequently, to a progression of endometriosis [33].

In comparison of urines samples of healthy patients with those with endometriosis, elevated levels of N1-metil-4-pyridone-5 carboxamide, guanidino-succinate, creatinine, taurine, valine and 2-hydroxyisovalerate were found in the samples of the endometriosis patients [17]. Most of these metabolites are involved in the inflammatory and oxidative stress process.

Cordeiro et al. decided to analyse the lipid profile in follicular fluid samples of patients who underwent in vitro fertilisation, concluding that levels of sphingolipids and phosphatidylcholines were higher in patients affected by endometriosis than in the control group [16].

Dominguez et al. used endometrial fluid samples of patients with endometriosis in their evaluation of a large panel of metabolites, finding reduced levels of sphingolipids monohexosylceramides and ceramides and higher levels of glycerophospholipids and glycerolipids [15].

Changes in sphingolipid metabolism have also been found in the peritoneal fluid, serum and endometrial tissue of patients with endometriosis [34]. These findings suggest that sphingolipids may play a crucial role in the pathogenesis of the disease and also have implications as potential biomarkers [15, 16, 19, 34].

## 2.4    Metabolomic Approach in Endometriosis: Therapeutic Perspectives

In addition to providing new biomarkers research for non-invasive diagnosis of endometriosis, metabolomics may be useful for identifying novel therapeutic strategies. Interesting perspectives on this have emerged from studies on glycerophospholipids and sphingolipids.

Different sphingomyelins were found in elevated concentrations in the plasma of patients affected by endometriosis [19]. The most plausible explanation for this phenomenon is the denervation, followed by reinnervation that occurs in the ectopic endometrium of these patients [35]. Sphingomyelins convert into sphingosine-1-phosphate (S1P), because of a change in the genetic expression of the enzymes involved in sphingomyelins' metabolic pathways. In fact, Borghese et al. showed that genes that encode enzymes that catalyse sphingomyelins conversion to S1P are upregulated in endometriotic tissue; on the other hand, genes that encode enzymes necessary to convert S1P to sphingosine are downregulated [36]. S1P promotes cell survival in response to apoptotic stimuli, thus explaining why endometriotic tissue is significantly less responsive to apoptosis versus healthy endometrial tissue [37]. Furthermore, Vouk et al. showed in their study that ether-phospholipids (three unsaturated 2-acyl-1-(1-alkenyl)-*sn*-glycerol-3-phosphocholines and two saturated 2-acyl-1-alkyl-*sn*-glycerol-3-phosphocholine) also reached high levels in endometriosis patients [19]. High concentrations of plasmanylcholines seem to be related to an increased request for platelet-activating factor (PAF) or PAF-like molecules in macrophages or neutrophils [38]. PAF is an inflammatory mediator, promoting, through its receptors, synthesis and release of neoangiogenic factors, like Vascular-Endothelial Growth Factor (VEGF). In the ectopic endometrial tissue, PAF synthesis increases due to major activity of various isoforms of the Phospholipase A2 (PLA-2) enzyme, which converts plasmacholines into lysoPAF, which is consequently converted into PAF by lysophosphatidylcholine-acyltransferase 4 (LPCAT4). This study suggests a possible new therapeutic strategy by inhibiting LPCAT4 and the hyper-expressed forms of PLA2 [19].

In conclusion, metabolomics could represent a powerful approach for finding novel diagnostic biomarkers through the analysis of the metabolic profile in endometriosis patients. Despite these results, metabolomics is not yet indicated as having enough specificity and sensitivity to distinguish disease cases from healthy controls; however, it might be useful for comprehending the pathogenetic mechanisms of a disease, and also as a way to discover other new therapeutic approaches.

## References

1. Angioni S. New insights on endometriosis. Minerva Ginecol. 2017;69:438–9. https://doi.org/10.23736/S0026-4784.17.04089-8.
2. Pontis A, Arena I, Angioni S. Umbilical endometriosis primary site without pelvic endometriosis and previous surgery: a case report. G Ital di Ostet e Ginecol. 2014;36:336–8. https://doi.org/10.11138/giog/2014.36.2.336.
3. Eisenberg VH, Weil C, Chodick G, Shalev V. Epidemiology of endometriosis: a large population-based database study from a healthcare provider with 2 million members. BJOG An Int J Obstet Gynaecol. 2018;125:55–62. https://doi.org/10.1111/1471-0528.14711.
4. Nisolle M, Donnez J. Peritoneal endometriosis, ovarian endometriosis, and adenomyotic nodules of the rectovaginal septum are three different entities. Fertil Steril. 1997;68:585–96. https://doi.org/10.1016/S0015-0282(97)00191-X.
5. Stochino-Loi E, Millochau J-C, Angioni S, Touleimat S, Abo C, Chanavaz-Lacheray I, Hennetier C, Roman H. Relationship between patient age and disease features in a prospective cohort of 1560 women affected by endometriosis. J Minim Invasive Gynecol. 2019;27:1158. https://doi.org/10.1016/j.jmig.2019.09.004.
6. Abrao MS, da C Gonçalves MO, Dias JA Jr, Podgaec S, Chamie LP, Blasbalg R. Comparison between clinical examination, transvaginal sonography and magnetic resonance imaging for the diagnosis of deep endometriosis. Hum Reprod. 2007;22:3092–7. https://doi.org/10.1093/humrep/dem187.
7. Dunselman GAJ, Vermeulen N, Becker C, Calhaz-Jorge C, D'Hooghe T, De Bie B, Heikinheimo O, Horne AW, Kiesel L, Nap A, Prentice A, Saridogan E, Soriano D, Nelen W, European Society of Human Reproduction and Embryology. ESHRE guideline: management of women with endometriosis. Hum Reprod. 2014;29:400–12. https://doi.org/10.1093/humrep/det457.
8. Antonio Maiorana. When more is not better: 10 "Don'ts" in endometriosis management. An ETIC * position statement. Hum Reprod Open. 2019; https://doi.org/10.1093/HROPEN/HOZ009.
9. Barbieri RL, Niloff JM, Bast RC, Scaetzl E, Kistner RW, Knapp RC. Elevated serum concentrations of CA-125 in patients with advanced endometriosis. Fertil Steril. 1986;45:630–4. https://doi.org/10.1016/S0015-0282(16)49333-7.
10. Socolov R, Butureanu S, Angioni S, Sindilar A, Boiculese L, Cozma L, Socolov D. The value of serological markers in the diagnosis and prognosis of endometriosis: a prospective case-control study. Eur J Obstet Gynecol Reprod Biol. 2011;154:215–7. https://doi.org/10.1016/j.ejogrb.2010.10.008.
11. Dutta M, Singh B, Joshi M, Das D, Subramani E, Maan M, Jana SK, Sharma U, Das S, Dasgupta S, Ray CD, Chakravarty B, Chaudhury K. Metabolomics reveals perturbations in endometrium and serum of minimal and mild endometriosis. Sci Rep. 2018;8:6466. https://doi.org/10.1038/s41598-018-23954-7.
12. Komala NT, Gurumurthy R, Surendra P. OMICS technologies towards seed quality improvement. Int J Pure App Biosci. 2017;5:1075–85. https://doi.org/10.18782/2320-7051.3072.
13. Nicholson JK, Lindon JC. Systems biology: metabonomics. Nature. 2008;455:1054–6. https://doi.org/10.1038/4551054a.

14. Emwas A-HM. The strengths and weaknesses of NMR spectroscopy and mass spectrometry with particular focus on metabolomics research. Methods Mol Biol. 2015;1277:161–93. https://doi.org/10.1007/978-1-4939-2377-9_13.

15. Domínguez F, Ferrando M, Díaz-Gimeno P, Quintana F, Fernández G, Castells I, Simón C. Lipidomic profiling of endometrial fluid in women with ovarian endometriosis. Biol Reprod. 2017;96:772–9. https://doi.org/10.1093/biolre/iox014.

16. Cordeiro FB, Cataldi TR, Perkel KJ, do Vale Teixeira da Costa L, Rochetti RC, Stevanato J, Eberlin MN, Zylbersztejn DS, Cedenho AP, Lo Turco EG. Lipidomics analysis of follicular fluid by ESI-MS reveals potential biomarkers for ovarian endometriosis. J Assist Reprod Genet. 2015;32:1817–25. https://doi.org/10.1007/s10815-015-0592-1.

17. Vicente-Muñoz S, Morcillo I, Puchades-Carrasco L, Payá V, Pellicer A, Pineda-Lucena A. Nuclear magnetic resonance metabolomic profiling of urine provides a noninvasive alternative to the identification of biomarkers associated with endometriosis. Fertil Steril. 2015;104:1202–9. https://doi.org/10.1016/j.fertnstert.2015.07.1149.

18. Dutta M, Joshi M, Srivastava S, Lodh I, Chakravarty B, Chaudhury K. A metabonomics approach as a means for identification of potential biomarkers for early diagnosis of endometriosis. Mol BioSyst. 2012;8:3281–7. https://doi.org/10.1039/c2mb25353d.

19. Vouk K, Hevir N, Ribić-Pucelj M, Haarpaintner G, Scherb H, Osredkar J, Möller G, Prehn C, Rižner TL, Adamski J. Discovery of phosphatidylcholines and sphingomyelins as biomarkers for ovarian endometriosis. Hum Reprod. 2012;27:2955–65. https://doi.org/10.1093/humrep/des152.

20. Li J, Guan L, Zhang H, Gao Y, Sun J, Gong X, Li D, Chen P, Liang X, Huang M, Bi H. Endometrium metabolomic profiling reveals potential biomarkers for diagnosis of endometriosis at minimal-mild stages. Reprod Biol Endocrinol. 2018;16:42. https://doi.org/10.1186/s12958-018-0360-z.

21. Lousse J-C, Defrère S, Colette S, Van Langendonckt A, Donnez J. Expression of eicosanoid biosynthetic and catabolic enzymes in peritoneal endometriosis. Hum Reprod. 2009;25:734–41. https://doi.org/10.1093/humrep/dep408.

22. As-Sanie S, Kim J, Schmidt-Wilcke T, Sundgren PC, Clauw DJ, Napadow V, Harris RE. Functional connectivity is associated with altered brain chemistry in women with endometriosis-associated chronic pelvic pain. J Pain. 2016;17:1–13. https://doi.org/10.1016/j.jpain.2015.09.008.

23. Liu H, Lang JH. Is abnormal eutopic endometrium the cause of endometriosis? The role of eutopic endometrium in pathogenesis of endometriosis. Med Sci Monit. 2011;17:92–9. https://doi.org/10.12659/MSM.881707.

24. Hayrabedyan S, Kyurkchiev S, Kehayov I. Endoglin (cd105) and S100A13 as markers of active angiogenesis in endometriosis. Reprod Biol. 2005;5:51–67.

25. Griffin JL, Shockcor JP. Metabolic profiles of cancer cells. Nat Rev Cancer. 2004;4:551–61. https://doi.org/10.1038/nrc1390.

26. Swanson MG, Vigneron DB, Tabatabai ZL, Males RG, Schmitt L, Carroll PR, James JK, Hurd RE, Kurhanewicz J. Proton HR-MAS spectroscopy and quantitative pathologic analysis of MRI/3D-MRSI-targeted postsurgical prostate tissues. Magn Reson Med. 2003;50:944–54. https://doi.org/10.1002/mrm.10614.

27. Tripathi P, Kamarajan P, Somashekar BS, MacKinnon N, Chinnaiyan AM, Kapila YL, Rajendiran TM, Ramamoorthy A. Delineating metabolic signatures of head and neck squamous cell carcinoma: phospholipase A2, a potential therapeutic target. Int J Biochem Cell Biol. 2012;44:1852–61. https://doi.org/10.1016/j.biocel.2012.06.025.

28. Schwickert G, Walenta S, Mueller-Klieser W, Sundfør K, Rofstad EK. Correlation of high lactate levels in human cervical Cancer with incidence of metastasis. Cancer Res. 1995;55:4757–9.

29. Hilvo M, De Santiago I, Gopalacharyulu P, Schmitt WD, Budczies J, Kuhberg M, Dietel M, Aittokallio T, Markowetz F, Denkert C, Sehouli J, Frezza C, Darb-Esfahani S, Braicu EI. Accumulated metabolites of hydroxybutyric acid serve as diagnostic and prognostic

biomarkers of ovarian high-grade serous carcinomas. Cancer Res. 2016;76:796–804. https://doi.org/10.1158/0008-5472.CAN-15-2298.

30. Dionyssopoulou E, Vassiliadis S, Evangeliou A, Koumantakis EE, Athanassakis I. Constitutive or induced elevated levels of L-carnitine correlate with the cytokine and cellular profile of endometriosis. J Reprod Immunol. 2005;65:159–70. https://doi.org/10.1016/j.jri.2004.12.002.

31. Hashim HA. Potential role of aromatase inhibitors in the treatment of endometriosis. Int J Women's Health. 2014;6:671–80. https://doi.org/10.2147/IJWH.S34684.

32. Huhtinen K, Desai R, Stahle M, Salminen A, Handelsman DJ, Perheentupa A, Poutanen M. Endometrial and endometriotic concentrations of estrone and estradiol are determined by local metabolism rather than circulating levels. J Clin Endocrinol Metab. 2012;97:4228–35. https://doi.org/10.1210/jc.2012-1154.

33. Ghazi N, Arjmand M, Akbari Z, Mellati AO, Saheb-Kashaf H, Zamani Z. H NMR- based metabolomics approaches as non-invasive tools for diagnosis of endometriosis. Int J Reprod Biomed. 2016;14:1–8.

34. Lee YH, Tan CW, Venkatratnam A, Tan CS, Cui L, Loh SF, Griffith L, Tannenbaum SR, Chan JKY. Dysregulated sphingolipid metabolism in endometriosis. J Clin Endocrinol Metab. 2014;99:E1913–21. https://doi.org/10.1210/jc.2014-1340.

35. Quinn M. Endometriosis: the consequence of neurological dysfunction? Med Hypotheses. 2004;63:602–8. https://doi.org/10.1016/j.mehy.2004.03.032.

36. Borghese B, Mondon F, Noël JC, Fayt I, Mignot TM, Vaiman D, Chapron C. Gene expression profile for ectopic versus eutopic endometrium provides new insights into endometriosis oncogenic potential. Mol Endocrinol. 2008;22:2557–62. https://doi.org/10.1210/me.2008-0322.

37. Gebel MH, Braun DP, Tambur A, Frame D, Rana N, Dmowski WP. Spontaneous apoptosis of endometrial tissue is impaired in women with endometriosis. Fertil Steril. 1998;69:1042–7. https://doi.org/10.1016/S0015-0282(98)00073-9.

38. Nagan N, Zoeller RA. Plasmalogens: biosynthesis and functions. Prog Lipid Res. 2001;40:199–229. https://doi.org/10.1016/S0163-7827(01)00003-0.

# Can We Diagnose Early Endometriosis with Ultrasound Rather than Laparoscopy?

Steven R. Goldstein

Endometriosis is defined by the World Endometriosis Society as an inflammatory condition characterized by endometrium-like tissue at sites outside the uterus [1]. Endometriosis afflicts 10% of women of reproductive age and 35–50% of women with pelvic pain or infertility [2]. It is classified either as superficial or as deeply infiltrating endometriosis (DIE) when the endometriotic tissue penetrates the retroperitoneal space for a distance of 5 mm or more. Endometriosis may present in multiple locations in the pelvis including the uterus (adenomyosis), ovary (endometrioma), pelvic peritoneum, bladder/ureter, rectum, colon, uterosacral ligaments, rectovaginal septum, vaginal wall, and pouch of Douglas.

Pain, a frequent symptom of endometriosis that manifests as dysmenorrhea, chronic pelvic pain, dyspareunia, and/or dyschezia, can be debilitating. Even among women without extensive disease, pain can limit daily life activities and negatively affect health-related quality of life and productivity, with substantial economic consequences [3]. The other major sequela of endometriosis is infertility that, for some women, is the only indicator of the disease. Endometriosis is detected among approximately 20–50% of women who undergo treatment for infertility and who do not present with symptoms such as pain or menstrual irregularities [4].

The profound influence of untreated endometriosis on many aspects of women's lives underscores the need for timely diagnosis and initiation of treatment. Nonetheless, diagnostic challenges coupled with the previous requirement for surgical intervention to make a diagnosis often result in considerable delay in the clinical management of affected individuals. Studies that have evaluated the timing of diagnosis in various parts of the world have consistently reported a mean or median

S. R. Goldstein (✉)
Obstetrics and Gynecology, New York University School of Medicine, New York, NY, USA

Gynecologic Ultrasound, Bone Densitometry, New York University Langone Medical Center, New York, NY, USA
e-mail: Steven.goldstein@nyulangone.org

© International Society of Gynecological Endocrinology 2021
A. R. Genazzani et al. (eds.), *Endometriosis Pathogenesis, Clinical Impact and Management*, ISGE Series, https://doi.org/10.1007/978-3-030-57866-4_3

interval of at least 7 years from the time a patient first experiences symptoms of endometriosis until she receives a confirmed diagnosis [5, 6]. In the interim, many women with endometriosis undergo consultations with multiple practitioners and receive misdiagnoses (e.g., chronic pelvic pain syndrome, idiopathic sterility, or pelvic inflammatory disease) before finally reaching the correct diagnosis [5].

The best methods to diagnose endometriosis and to determine the extent and pathologic severity of this disease are subject to debate [4]. A recent review still stated, "The only reliable diagnosis of endometriosis today is diagnostic laparoscopy with inspection of the abdominal cavity and histological confirmation of suspect lesions" [2]. The need for histological confirmation nevertheless remains debatable as macroscopically recognized endometriotic lesions are not always histologically confirmed. Conversely, occult microscopic endometriosis can be detected in biopsies of macroscopically normal peritoneum of women with and without visible endometriosis [7].

Any discussion of the diagnosis of endometriosis must begin by defining what constitutes this disease. Endometriosis is traditionally defined by the presence of lesions, which vary considerably in appearance, size, and location, and are histologically confirmed by the detection of endometrial glands, endometrial stroma, and/or hemosiderin-laden macrophages. However, an internationally accepted definition proposed in 2017 describes endometriosis as "a disease characterized by the presence of endometrium-like epithelium and stroma outside the endometrium and myometrium. Intrapelvic endometriosis can be located superficially on the peritoneum (peritoneal endometriosis), can extend 5 mm or more beneath the peritoneum (deep endometriosis), or can be present as an ovarian endometriotic cyst (endometrioma)" [8]. These definitions are based solely on pathology and do not consider symptoms such as pain and infertility that act as drivers for the initiation of treatment. The ability to diagnose endometriosis clinically requires a different approach in which symptoms are considered to be paramount and histology is a secondary criterion.

In the past visualization—typically by laparoscopy with histologic confirmation—is generally considered to be the gold standard (Table 3.1) [4, 9–12]. However, this technique is not without its limitations, costs, and risks. In practice, clinicians often rely on medical history, presenting symptoms, and findings on physical examination (i.e., a clinical diagnosis), with or without imaging studies, as the basis for initiating therapy. This practice is consistent with guidance from the American College of Obstetricians and Gynecologists [4], the Society of Obstetricians and Gynaecologists of Canada [10], the European Society of Human Reproduction and Embryology [4] (also endorsed by the Royal College of Obstetricians and Gynaecologists), and the World Endometriosis Society (WES) [12]. These organizations advocate for empiric treatment before laparoscopy in selected patients (Table 3.1) [4, 9–12]. The American Society for Reproductive Medicine (ASRM) guidelines state that laparoscopy before empiric treatment is the "preferred approach, although further studies are warranted" (Table 3.1) [9].

**Table 3.1** Summary of key recommendations regarding the diagnosis and treatment of endometriosis

| Method of diagnosis | ACOG | ASRM | SOGC | ESHRE | WES |
|---|---|---|---|---|---|
| Clinical | Definitive diagnosis can only be made by surgery with histologic verification | Laparoscopy before empiric treatment is the "preferred approach, although further studies are warranted" | "Investigation of suspected endometriosis should include patient history, physical examination, and imaging studies" | "The diagnosis of endometriosis is suspected based on the history, the symptoms and signs, is corroborated by physical examination and imaging techniques and is finally proven by histological examination of specimens collected during laparoscopy" | Diagnostic gold standard is laparoscopic visualization, preferably with histologic confirmation |
| | Empiric treatment can be offered before diagnostic laparoscopy, although a response to therapy does not confirm the diagnosis | Operative visualization can be an acceptable surrogate to histologic diagnosis in some cases, although atypical lesions are difficult to characterize without biopsy | Direct visualization at laparoscopy with histologic verification is the gold standard; however, empiric treatment can be offered before diagnostic laparoscopy | Empiric treatment for pain can be offered before diagnostic laparoscopy | Empiric medical therapy can be initiated before surgical diagnosis and treatment but should be preceded by a full evaluation |
| TVUS | Preferred imaging technique when assessing endometriosis and/or deep endometriosis of the rectum or rectovaginal septum | Imaging modalities have not been found to increase diagnostic accuracy | "First-line investigational tool for suspected endometriosis" | "Useful for identifying or ruling out rectal endometriosis" | Not discussed |
| | | | | Recommended to diagnose or exclude ovarian endometrioma | |

(continued)

**Table 3.1** (continued)

| Method of diagnosis | ACOG | ASRM | SOGC | ESHRE | WES |
|---|---|---|---|---|---|
| MRI | Reserved for suspected rectovaginal or bladder endometriosis when ultrasonographic results are equivocal | Imaging modalities have not been found to increase diagnostic accuracy | Could be required if deep endometriosis is suspected | Usefulness for diagnosing peritoneal endometriosis is not well-established | Not discussed |

Abbreviations: *ACOG* American College of Obstetricians and Gynecologists, *ASRM* American Society for Reproductive Medicine, *SOGC* Society of Obstetricians and Gynaecologists of Canada, *ESHRE* European Society of Human Reproduction and Embryology, *WES* World Endometriosis Society, *TVUS* Transvaginal ultrasonography, *MRI* magnetic resonance imaging
Reproduced with permission. *Credit:* Taylor, H.S., Adamson, G.D., Diamond M.P., Goldstein, S.R., Horne, A.W., Missmer, S.A., Snabes, M.C., Surrey E. and Taylor, R.N. (2018), An evidence-based approach to assessing surgical versus clinical diagnosis of symptomatic endometriosis. Int J Gynecol Obstet, 142: 131–142. doi:https://doi.org/10.1002/ijgo.12521. *Creator:* © 2018 The Authors. International Journal of Gynecology & Obstetrics published by John Wiley & Sons Ltd. on behalf of International Federation of Gynecology and Obstetrics

## 3.1    Clinical Diagnosis of Endometriosis

Clinical presentations of endometriosis are highly diverse; none of the presenting signs or symptoms are pathognomonic for this disease. Because of the overlap in symptoms with other gynecologic conditions (e.g., primary dysmenorrhea, adenomyosis, pelvic adhesions, ovarian cysts, pelvic inflammatory disease) and chronic pain syndromes (e.g., irritable bowel, interstitial cystitis/painful bladder, fibromyalgia, musculoskeletal disorders), differential diagnosis is an important facet of identifying endometriosis. By way of example, gynecologic conditions such as primary dysmenorrhea, adenomyosis, pelvic adhesions, ovarian cysts, and pelvic inflammatory disease should be excluded, as should chronic pain syndromes, including irritable bowel, interstitial cystitis, painful bladder, fibromyalgia, and musculoskeletal disorders.

Pelvic pain is a common occurrence among the general population. Although pain is a cardinal symptom of endometriosis, discerning whether it can be attributed to endometriosis is challenging. Pelvic pain among women can arise from a variety of sources and have multiple presentations and characteristics, which complicates its value as a marker of endometriosis. Dysmenorrhea, chronic pelvic pain, chronic nonmenstrual pelvic pain, and dyspareunia are the most consistently reported types of pain among women with endometriosis [13–17]. Overall, dysmenorrhea is the most frequent pain symptom, reported by the majority of women who have proven endometriosis. Chronic pelvic pain and/or chronic nonmenstrual pelvic pain are generally less common than dysmenorrhea but are notable for their higher occurrence rates in women with proven or self-reported endometriosis than in women without endometriosis [13].

Women with endometriosis typically experience pain. Although the occurrence of pelvic pain alone is insufficient to diagnose endometriosis or to categorize the type or stage of the disease, certain characteristics (e.g., dysmenorrhea, progression, and insufficient response to NSAIDs or oral contraceptives) may be indicative of endometriosis.

### 3.1.1    Physical Examination

Multiple studies have sought to quantify the ability of a physical examination to detect endometriosis by gauging its accuracy relative to surgical diagnosis [16, 18–20]. Patient selection and examination methods differ among individual studies, which confound the overall estimation of accuracy.

### 3.1.2    Ultrasonography

So, how can we improve non-surgical diagnosis beyond pain and/or clinical findings? Imaging methods such as ultrasonography have inherent value for their ability to identify causes of abdominal pain and menstrual symptoms other than endometriosis (e.g., adenomyosis). In the context of endometriosis, the addition of transvaginal ultrasonography (TVUS) to pelvic examination increases the accuracy of a clinical diagnosis of adnexal and rectal disease [21]. Hudelist et al. [21] reported almost universal increases in the sensitivity of endometriosis detection when TVUS was combined with pelvic examination versus pelvic examination alone among women with symptoms suggestive of endometriosis. Of note, sensitivity for detecting ovarian endometriosis increased from approximately 30% with pelvic examination alone to greater than 96% with pelvic examination plus TVUS.

A strong correlation has been observed between TVUS markers and laparoscopic findings. Among 120 consecutive women with chronic pelvic pain evaluated by Okaro et al. [22], "hard markers" on TVUS (structural abnormalities such as endometriomas or hydrosalpinges) demonstrated a 100% correlation (24 of 24 women) with laparoscopic findings. In addition, "soft" markers (e.g., reduced ovarian mobility, site-specific pelvic tenderness, and the presence of loculated peritoneal fluid in the pelvis) were predictive of pelvic pathology, with 37 of 51 (73%) of women with only soft markers by TVUS having a true-positive result. These data lend support to an empiric course of treatment, as 61 of 75 (81%) women evaluated by TVUS had their need for treatment confirmed laparoscopically.

There are some limitations when considering an ultrasound capability of making a presumptive diagnosis of endometriosis with high enough predictive value to warrant medical therapy without laparoscopy. In some parts of the world, ultrasound is performed as an imaging examination by trained imagers, often employing sonographers (also known as technicians) to do the scans and image capture. The images are then often read as static images or, occasionally, video clips after the study is complete. The increasing use of remote teleradiology further compounds this methodology.

### 3.1.3   Dynamic Ultrasound

Hence, the concept of dynamic ultrasound. Gynecologic healthcare providers have used the bimanual exam for diagnosis for decades. When one thinks of such an exam, it really consists of two components. The first, the objective component, tries to assess anatomic features such as—Is the uterus enlarged or not? Is it irregular in contour suggesting leiomyomas? Is the ovary normal sized and, if not, does it feel cystic or solid? Such anatomy may be replaced in a matter of minutes with imaging if one has sufficient skill and equipment. The second component of the bimanual exam is that of a subjective nature—is there tenderness, is there normal mobility? This cannot be replaced with an image. This requires the experience and nuance of the examiner.

There is an inherent difference between an ultrasound examination, as it is often performed by referral to a dedicated imager and this concept of examining one's patients with ultrasound. This new concept of dynamic ultrasound implies that anyone performing imaging must also *examine* the patient, either with the movement of the probe or the other hand on the lower abdomen. This is done to see if there is normal mobility or tenderness. This is the kind of ultrasound assessment used in the study by Okaro et al. [22]. Such a concept was originated by Timor [23] as the sliding organ sign. Obviously, the presence of a classic endometrioma has virtually 100% sensitivity for non-laparoscopic diagnosis of endometriosis. However, if one employs dynamic scanning, and the work by Okaro et al. [22] is duplicated by further studies, one can expect that 73% of the endometriosis can be diagnosed by such dynamic ultrasound scanning. Clearly, further study is necessary.

In summary, endometriosis can be a tremendous source of pain and/or infertility. In the past and still, some healthcare providers believe the only definitive diagnosis is by laparoscopy. However, there is evidence that the use of dynamic ultrasound and understanding of "soft markers," holds great promise to make a presumptive diagnosis of high enough probability to warrant medical therapy without laparoscopy.

## References

1. Johnson NP, Hummelshoj L, Adamson GD, et al. World endometriosis society consensus on the classification of endometriosis. Hum Reprod. 2017;32:315–24.
2. Kiesel L, Sourouni M. Diagnosis of endometriosis in the 21st century. Climacteric. 2019;22:296–302.
3. Nnoaham KE, Hummelshoj L, Webster P, et al. Impact of endometriosis on quality of life and work productivity: a multicenter study across ten countries. Fertil Steril. 2011;96:366–73.
4. American College of Obstetricians and Gynecologists. Practice bulletin no. 114: management of endometriosis. Obstet Gynecol. 2010;116:223–36. (Reaffirmed 2018).
5. Hudelist G, Fritzer N, Thomas A, et al. Diagnostic delay for endometriosis in Austria and Germany: causes and possible consequences. Hum Reprod. 2012;27:3412–6.
6. Staal AH, van der Zanden M, Nap AW. Diagnostic delay of endometriosis in the Netherlands. Gynecol Obstet Investig. 2016;81:321–4.
7. Hopton EN, Redwine DB. Eyes wide shut: the illusory tale of 'occult' microscopic endometriosis. Hum Reprod. 2014;29:384–7.
8. Zegers-Hochschild F, Adamson GD, Dyer S, et al. The international glossary on infertility and fertility care, 2017. Fertil Steril. 2017;108:393–406.
9. Practice Committee of the American Society for Reproductive Medicine. Treatment of pelvic pain associated with endometriosis: a committee opinion. Fertil Steril. 2014;101:927–35.
10. Leyland N, Casper R, Laberge P, Singh SS, the Society of Obstetricians and Gynaecologists of Canada. Endometriosis: diagnosis and management. J Obstet Gynaecol Can. 2010;32:S1–S32.
11. Dunselman GA, Vermeulen N, Becker C, et al. ESHRE guideline: management of women with endometriosis. Hum Reprod. 2014;29:400–12.
12. Johnson NP, Hummelshoj L, world endometriosis society Montpellier C. Consensus on current management of endometriosis. Hum Reprod. 2013;28:1552–68.
13. Schliep KC, Mumford SL, Peterson CM, et al. Pain typology and incident endometriosis. Hum Reprod. 2015;30:2427–38.
14. Apostolopoulos NV, Alexandraki KI, Gorry A, Coker A. Association between chronic pelvic pain symptoms and the presence of endometriosis. Arch Gynecol Obstet. 2016;293:439–45.
15. Ballard KD, Seaman HE, de Vries CS, Wright JT. Can symptomatology help in the diagnosis of endometriosis? Findings from a national case-control study—part 1. BJOG. 2008;115:1382–91.
16. Eskenazi B, Warner M, Bonsignore L, Olive D, Samuels S, Vercellini P. Validation study of nonsurgical diagnosis of endometriosis. Fertil Steril. 2001;76:929–35.
17. Porpora MG, Koninckx PR, Piazze J, Natili M, Colagrande S, Cosmi EV. Correlation between endometriosis and pelvic pain. J Am Assoc Gynecol Laparosc. 1999;6:429–34.

18. Hudelist G, Ballard K, English J, et al. Transvaginal sonography vs. clinical examination in the preoperative diagnosis of deep infiltrating endometriosis. Ultrasound Obstet Gynecol. 2011;37:480–7.
19. Abrao MS, Goncalves MO, Dias JA Jr, Podgaec S, Chamie LP, Blasbalg R. Comparison between clinical examination, transvaginal sonography and magnetic resonance imaging for the diagnosis of deep endometriosis. Hum Reprod. 2007;22:3092–7.
20. Cheewadhanaraks S, Peeyananjarassri K, Dhanaworavibul K, Liabsuetrakul T. Positive predictive value of clinical diagnosis of endometriosis. J Med Assoc Thail. 2004;87:740–4.
21. Hudelist G, Oberwinkler KH, Singer CF, et al. Combination of transvaginal sonography and clinical examination for preoperative diagnosis of pelvic endometriosis. Hum Reprod. 2009;24:1018–24.
22. Okaro E, Condous G, Khalid A, et al. The use of ultrasound-based 'soft markers' for the prediction of pelvic pathology in women with chronic pelvic pain–can we reduce the need for laparoscopy? BJOG. 2006;113:251–6.
23. Timor-Tritsch I. Sliding organs sign in gynecologic ultrasound. Ultrasound Obstet Gynecol. 2015;46:125–6.

# Neurotrophins and Cytokines in Endometriosis Pain

# 4

Robert N. Taylor, Jie Yu, Antônio M. C. Francisco, Sarah L. Berga, and Dan I. Lebovic

## 4.1    Introduction

Endometriosis is a gynecological syndrome associated with pain and infertility and characterized by the growth of hormoneresponsive endometrial tissue outside the uterine cavity. Recent population-based estimates put its overall frequency among reproductive-age women at around 11%; hence, it afflicts millions of women worldwide, resulting in work absenteeism, social isolation, and high costs of medical and surgical therapies. In this chapter, the authors offer hypotheses as to the role of "neuroangiogenesis" in endometriosis pathogenesis and pathophysiology. Mediators of lesion-associated pain and current and future therapeutic strategies are offered. Evolution of our understanding about the biology of this chronic disease promises to expand treatment choices for women suffering from its complications.

R. N. Taylor (✉)
Department of Obstetrics and Gynecology, University of Utah School of Medicine, Salt Lake City, UT, USA

Department of Obstetrics and Gynecology, Wake Forest School of Medicine, Winston-Salem, NC, USA
e-mail: Rob.taylor@hsc.utah.edu

J. Yu
Department of Obstetrics and Gynecology, Wake Forest School of Medicine, Winston-Salem, NC, USA

A. M. C. Francisco
Faculdade de Ciências da Saúde, Universidade do Vale do Sapucaí, Pouso Alegre, Minas Gerais, Brazil

S. L. Berga
Department of Obstetrics and Gynecology, University of Utah School of Medicine, Salt Lake City, UT, USA

D. I. Lebovic
Center for Reproductive Medicine, Minneapolis, MN, USA

© International Society of Gynecological Endocrinology 2021
A. R. Genazzani et al. (eds.), *Endometriosis Pathogenesis, Clinical Impact and Management*, ISGE Series, https://doi.org/10.1007/978-3-030-57866-4_4

## 4.2    Clinical Presentation

Endometriosis has been identified in women ranging in age from 12 to 80, with an average of ~28 years old. Exposure to ovarian hormones appears to be essential to stimulating lesion growth. Although its precise mechanisms remain mysterious, the most common symptom in women with endometriosis is progressive, secondary dysmenorrhea. The pain typically begins before menses and continues throughout the duration of menstrual flow. It may be accompanied by dyspareunia, dysuria, dyschezia, or noncyclic pelvic pain [3]. The pain also may be referred to musculo-skeletal regions, such as the flank or low back.

Due to the pusillanimous, diffuse nature of common parietal peritoneal endometriosis lesions, physical examination can be unremarkable. However, the astute clinician can sometimes appreciate pain or induration with palpation in the vicinity of the cul-de-sac or rectovaginal septum. Tender nodules along the uterosacral ligaments, especially if the examination is done just before menses, can sometimes be identified. Rarely, impaired renal function and azotemia can occur in women with retroperitoneal ureteric fibrosis that compromises urinary drainage.

Cyclic in situ menstruation at the sites of endometriotic lesions is thought to activate a chronic inflammatory response involving cytokine release and prostaglandin biosynthesis, leading to pain perception. In some cases, direct infiltration of endometriotic cells into afferent nerves has been observed [4]. Furthermore, the enhanced inflammatory milieu may result in sensitization of dorsal root ganglia and central neurons [5]. New hypotheses suggest that coordinated neural and vascular growth, "neuroangiogenesis," and secondary central neuropathic sequelae contribute to pelvic pain [6, 7].

## 4.3    Genomics, Genetics, and Epigenetics

Genes strongly influence susceptibility for endometriosis [8] and its heritability is estimated to be as high as 51%. However, the mode of transmission is polygenic and involves multiple gene loci [9]. Early evidence indicated that first-degree female relatives (mothers and sisters) of women with severe endometriosis had a 7% incidence, whereas in primary female relatives of their partners (who typically have similar ethnic and socioeconomic status) <1% had endometriosis [10]. Of interest is the finding that familial cases of endometriosis tend to be more severe and have an earlier onset of symptoms than sporadic cases. Endocrine disruptor compounds in the environment are thought to affect endometriosis, a subject that is presented in Chap. 1 by Palumbo and colleagues.

## 4.4    Pathogenesis

Descriptions of the symptoms and pathological features of endometriosis date back to Dutch and Belgian publications of the 1600s [11]. The great German pathologists Karl von Rokitansky and Robert Meyer wrote extensively about this disorder in the nineteenth century, and the Canadian physician, Thomas Cullen, is credited for identifying endometriosis as a unique disease in the 1890s. In the 1920s an American gynecologist named John Sampson put forward the hypothesis that pelvic endometriosis lesions arose from endometrial tissue escaping through the fallopian tubes at the time of menstruation. Viable tissue fragments, he postulated, implanted on and invaded peritoneal surfaces, where they regenerated an endometrial epithelial lining [12].

### 4.4.1    Retrograde Menstruation, Implantation, and Lesion Establishment

Still today, the prevailing hypothesis concerning the histogenesis of endometriosis is Sampson's implantation theory [12]. This concept is supported by the visual documentation of reflux menstruation [13], intraperitoneal spillage of competent endometrial cells, and the gravity-dependent location of most foci of endometriosis. Furthermore, the incidence is increased in women with Müllerian anomalies and menstrual outflow obstruction [14]. Finally, more than 60% of unilateral ureteral endometriosis lesions occur in the left hemipelvis, which is consistent with the accumulation of refluxed cells in this location, due to the position of the sigmoid colon mesentery [15].

Although some controversy exists as to whether or not lesion implantation requires a breach in the mesothelial surface or if endometriosis cells are capable of invading intact mesothelium, the expression of adhesion molecules on the surface of exfoliated uterine cells is thought to be necessary for nascent lesion attachment and invasion [16]. Cytokines (e.g., interleukin (IL)-1β, IL-6, and tumor necrosis factor (TNF)-α) and relative steroid hormone sensitivity predispose the adhesion of shed endometrial fragments, facilitating peritoneal invasion.

### 4.4.2    Angiogenic Factors

Implantation of ectopic endometrium sets into motion a step-wise pathophysiological program involving hormone responsiveness and immune cell activation, as depicted in Fig. 4.1. How these progressive interactions appear to promote the establishment of endometriosis lesions is addressed in this review. Given the universality of retrograde menstruation [13], it is not clear why endometriosis affects only ~11% of women. It is postulated that the intrinsic angiogenic potential of the intraperitoneal environment dictates the likelihood of lesion establishment. At laparoscopy, endometriotic implants are often surrounded by exaggerated vascularity

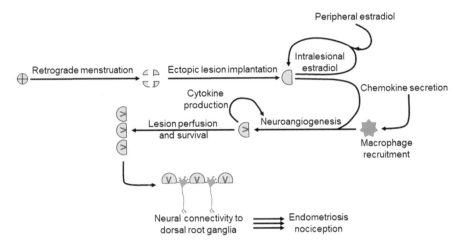

**Fig. 4.1** Proposed, step-wise establishment of nascent peritoneal endometriotic implants via retrograde menstruation, attachment, proliferation, migration, inflammation, neovascularization, neurogenesis, and fibrosis, leading to pain

and in the rare occurrence of extrapelvic endometriosis, it is often localized in well-vascularized sites.

Sprouting angiogenesis of new blood vessels from preexisting capillaries is a complex process involving proteolytic degradation of the extracellular matrix, proliferation, and migration of endothelial cells, and ultimately the organization of cell columns into patent capillary tubules. Many angiogenic growth factors and cytokines have been identified in endometriosis and reviewed recently [17]. Vascular endothelial growth factor (VEGF) is primary among those proteins; moreover, it also has neurogenic properties [6]. VEGF is known to be an estrogen-responsive gene, particularly in the uterus [18].

### 4.4.3 Estrogen Biosynthesis, Receptors, and Action Are Critical for Endometriosis Lesion Growth

One of the defining characteristics of endometriosis is its endocrine responsiveness, particularly with respect to estrogen. Typically, endometriosis pain symptoms begin after the onset of menses and, in the majority of cases, resolve after menopause. The estrogen dependency of this condition led Barbieri to propose the hypothesis that concentrations of estradiol over 50 pg/mL were needed to support the growth of endometriosis lesions [19]. His hypothesis proved to be prescient as more recent and sophisticated pharmacometrics studies of a variety of gonadotropin-releasing hormone analog (GnRHa) drugs have revealed that a threshold of 30–50 pg/mL estradiol is highly correlated with endometriosis symptom recurrence in clinical trials [20]. Promising data are beginning to appear in the literature supporting the use of orally active GnRH antagonists for the treatment of endometriosis-associated pain and improvement in quality of life measures [3]. These therapeutic options will be discussed in more detail elsewhere in this monograph by De Villiers (Chap. 14). Body mass index (BMI) correlates inversely with the risk of endometriosis [21]. Other more sophisticated anthropometric assessment measurements (e.g., skin-fold thickness, arm, waist, chest and hip circumferences) failed to add more predictive power for endometriosis risk than low BMI.

Steroid biosynthesis and metabolism actively occur within these lesions, where an entire range of steroidogenic enzymes are expressed, including steroid acute regulatory (StAR) protein, cholesterol P450 side-chain cleavage, 3β-hydroxysteroid dehydrogenase type 2, 17α-hydroxylase and aromatase. Thus, endometriotic lesions have co-opted the ability to generate their own local estrogenic milieu using cholesterol as a substrate [22].

Like its derivative eutopic endometrium, endometriotic lesions express the gamut of nuclear steroid and isoprenoid receptors, as reviewed elsewhere [22, 23], which impart broad hormone responsivity to the implants. Moreover, the expression of some receptor isoforms differs from those in normal endometrium, providing a growth advantage to the ectopic foci. In particular, estrogen receptor β (ESR2) is highly expressed in endometriosis and concentrations of progesterone receptor B (PGR-B) are downregulated. An apparent epigenetic mechanism in the former case is a result of the hypomethylation of CpG islands in the *ESR2* gene promoter [24].

### 4.4.4 Innervation of Endometriosis Implants

The parietal peritoneum is richly innervated by somatic and visceral afferents arising from branches of the lower intercostal and upper lumbar nerves. Unmyelinated sensory Aδ- and C-nerve endings are exposed to nociceptive biochemical stimuli, which are perceived as sharp pain referred to the periumbilical, suprapubic, or lower abdominal regions. Interestingly, the visceral peritoneum has little innervation, but submesothelial autonomic nerves are present that respond to traction and pressure [25].

Anaf et al. [26] were among the first to postulate that pelvic pain arising from endometriosis might be associated with peritoneal nerve fibers. They observed that subjects with nodular lesions demonstrating perineural invasion had the highest pelvic pain scores. Tulandi et al. [27] used anti-neurofilament antibodies and immunohistochemistry methods to quantify nerve fiber density and neurofilament protein intensity but did not observe more nerves in peritoneal specimens from endometriosis subjects compared to women without endometriosis. Interestingly, in the latter study, they did note more "lymphocytic infiltration" in the histological samples from women with laparoscopically-proven endometriosis than controls. We will discuss this finding in more detail when we address the potential immune modulators of neuroangiogenesis in this setting.

A pioneering study in this field was performed not in women but in rats with surgically induced "endometriosis." Berkley and colleagues [28] autotransplanted uterine tissue fragments to the bowel mesentery and noted that after ~7.5 weeks, the cystic lesions of ectopic endometrium had acquired a rich plexus of nerves that immunostained positively for neuronal markers indicating the presence of sensory Aδ- and C-fibers along with sympathetic nerves. An additional observation at that time was that neurites growing out of these lesions were accompanied by a dense microvasculature. These findings further support the concept of lesion neuroangiogenesis proposed some years later [6].

By the 2000s, investigators were reporting histological evidence that nociceptive and autonomic afferent nerves were present in endometriotic lesions of women [29]. An important extension of this line of research, first announced by the Australian group [30] and confirmed by Belgian scientists [31], was the discovery that eutopic endometrium from women with endometriosis had a higher density of nerve fibers than the endometrium of unaffected controls. This topic has been argued in the literature, but many studies support neuron density as a distinguishing feature between women with and without endometriosis. As detailed in the introductory part of this chapter, such a finding is consistent with Sampson's implantation theory that ectopic lesions are derived from shed eutopic endometrium. The idea that eutopic endometrium is the "mother of the implants" in endometriosis is an important contemporary concept in the pathogenesis of this disorder [23].

If ectopic, and even eutopic, endometrial tissues in endometriosis are imbued with a higher density of nociceptive nerves than in unaffected women there must be some trophic factor responsible for this phenomenon. This was a question asked by a number of endometriosis scholars in the early 2000s. Borghese et al. [32] posed this question by assessing a panel of neurotrophin mRNAs in endometriomas and eutopic endometrium using reverse transcription-polymerase chain reaction methods. They reported that transcripts representing nerve growth factor (NGF), brain-derived growth factor (BDNF), neurotrophin-2, neurotrophin-4/5, and the neurotrophin receptor (NTRK2) were all greater in endometrioma samples than in eutopic endometrial tissues from the same subjects. Similar findings reported by Kajitani et al. [33] indicated that NGF mRNA levels were higher in endometrioma and peritoneal lesions than in normal endometrium. In studies from Belgium and France, endometriosis glands at the leading edge of deeply invasive lesions had elevated NGF, N-cadherin, and matrix metalloproteinase 9, and all were accompanied by a high density of nerves [34]. The density of protein gene product (PGP) 9.5-positive nerve fibers also was noted to be associated with deep dyspareunia in cases of endometriosis [35].

Our research team asked a slightly different question and used an agnostic, monoclonal antibody microarray method to compare the expression of neurotrophin proteins in eutopic endometria from women with or without surgically documented endometriosis. Our findings identified many of the same neurogenic factors described above, with BDNF, neurotrophin-3, and neurotrophin-4/5 being the predominant endometrial proteins differentially overexpressed in endometriosis cases [36]. Among these, BDNF concentrations were almost 1000-fold more enriched in endometrial lysates than the other neurotrophins. NGF was present in both sets of tissues but did not differ in concentration between the two patient groups. More recent studies have confirmed that even plasma concentrations of BDNF are increased in women with endometriosis and in some cases, these concentrations correlate with the severity of pelvic pain in affected subjects [37]; however, in most reports, the positive and negative predictive value of discriminating concentrations of BDNF and other biomarkers are not adequate for diagnostic testing or screening purposes [38].

One interesting biochemical aspect of these trophic factors, alluded to above, is that they possess both neurogenic and angiogenic activities. As noted above, the role of angiogenesis in the microenvironment of endometriosis lesions was established in the 1990s [39, 40]. Based on the tightly coupled growth of nerves and capillaries, e.g., during embryonic development and wound healing [41], we proposed that guidance molecules and their receptors common to nociceptive neurons and vascular endothelial cells were expressed in endometriosis tissues, allowing nascent implants to simultaneously recruit nerves and blood vessels through a cooperative process of neuroangiogenesis [6]. Several of these guidance proteins (e.g., BDNF, NGF, VEGF, semaphorin E) and their cognate receptors (e.g., TRK2, VEGFR1, Neuropilin, Plexin-D1, and Robo4 [42]) have been identified in endometriosis [43].

The peritoneal fluid that bathes the superficial lesions also has been identified as a source of neuroangiogenic factors. High levels of NGF were demonstrated in the pelvic fluid of endometriosis cases by Western blotting and its biological activity was confirmed by neurite outgrowth from chicken dorsal root ganglia in vitro. Some studies show correlations among peritoneal fluid cytokine concentrations, nerve fiber density, and pelvic pain [44], but these relationships do not hold true in all studies. In one report, pelvic pain scores were highest in subjects with histologically confirmed perineural invasion in deep endometriosis lesions, and these also demonstrated an increased density of neuroangiogenic activity [45]. A potential mechanism to promote neuroangiogenesis in the vicinity of endometriosis lesions is via exosome secretion. Exosomes derived from endometriosis subjects preferentially induced endothelial tube formation from primary human umbilical vein cells and neurite outgrowth from murine dorsal root ganglia in vitro [46, 47].

### 4.4.5 Endocrine and Cytokine Regulation of Neuroangiogenic Effects

Estrogenic and inflammatory influences are important modulators of nociception in endometriosis. Some effects are relatively direct; for example, in ovariectomized mice, administration of estradiol increased uterine BDNF and NGF receptor expression and NGF receptor mRNA levels also were upregulated [48]. In an established immunocompetent mouse model of endometriosis, we and our collaborators demonstrated that two selective estrogen receptor modulators (SERMs): oxabicycloheptene sulfonate (an ESR1 ligand) and chlorindazole (an ESR2 selective SERM), arrested cell proliferation, lesion growth, and neuroangiogenesis in surgically induced implants. This murine model corroborated that estrogens and macrophage-derived cytokines interact to promote the growth of peripheral nerves and emphasized that both isoforms of the ESR appear to have important actions on the establishment of endometriosis lesions [22].

Macrophages commonly infiltrate the microenvironment of endometriosis lesions. Strong evidence indicates that these inflammatory phagocytes are recruited to the implants by chemokines such as RANTES (CCL5) or MCP-1 (CCL2). Macrophage-derived cytokines, particularly IL-1β and TNF-α, are enriched in the peritoneal fluid of women with endometriosis [23]. IL-1β was found to directly stimulate BDNF mRNA and protein in endometriosis cell cultures, an effect that was predominantly mediated by c-Jun N-terminal kinase and nuclear factor κB (NF-κB) signaling pathways [49]. More recently, IGF-1 derived from macrophages also was shown to promote neurogenesis within the inflammatory foci of endometriosis implants [50]. Figure 4.2 provides an illustration of invasive endometriosis with classical glandular and stromal elements (panel A). Isolated macrophages, stained with anti-CD68 antibodies (magenta), have infiltrated the lesion (panel B) and BDNF is expressed by glands and stroma (panel C). In panel D, PGP9.5-positive nerve fibers (magenta) are viewed *en face* in the cut section, innervating the lesion. The regional confluence of endometriotic cells, immune cells, and nerve cells, along with capillaries (not shown in this tableau), supports the hypothesis that chemokines and neuroangiogenic factors produced in situ establish a microenvironment that recruits nociceptive nerves to the growing lesion, which we postulate ultimately effects endometriosis-associated pain.

### 4.4.6 Central Sensitization in Endometriosis-Associated Pain

Many of the experiments described in this review were designed to address how peripheral, peritoneal neuroangiogenesis can contribute to nociception of lesions in endometriosis, but another critical component of the processing of pain symptoms, particularly chronic pelvic pain, is mediated via central sensitization. Neuroimaging of the brain in 17 women with surgically confirmed endometriosis and chronic pelvic pain compared with 23 controls without pain revealed decreased grey matter volume in the left thalamus, left cingulate gyrus, right putamen, and right insula of the affected subjects; all four brain regions are known to be involved in pain processing [51]. The stress axis and other psychological factors also can modulate the perception of chronic pain, such that causes as well as consequences of pain and other somatic symptoms are associated with endometriosis [52].

### 4.5 Medical Therapy for Pain Associated with Endometriosis

Currently approved medications for endometriosis pain, endorsed by the U.S. Food and Drug Administration (FDA) or the European Medicines Agency (EMEA) include progestins (depot medroxyprogesterone acetate, norethindrone acetate, and dienogest), an androgen (danazol), and GnRHa. In 2018 the FDA also approved the oral GnRH antagonist elagolix for moderate to severe endometriosis pain. In

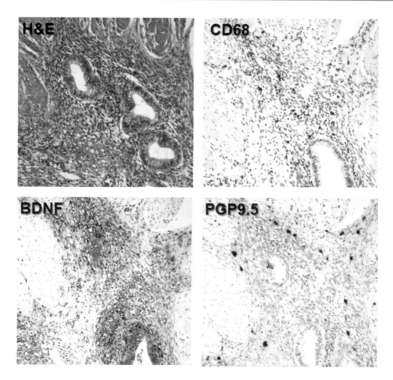

**Fig. 4.2** Endometriosis lesion stained with hematoxylin and eosin (upper left panel), CD68 (anti-macrophage) (upper right panel), BDNF (anti-neurotrophin) (lower left panel), and PGP9.5 (anti-nerve fibers) (lower right panel). Note that nerve fibers in the lower middle panel are mostly viewed en face relative to the orientation of the implant. Magnification × 200. (Reproduced with permission from Yu J, Francisco AMC, Patel BG, Cline JM, Zou E, Berga SL and Taylor RN. IL-1β stimulates BDNF production in eutopic endometriosis stromal cell cultures: A model for cytokine regulation of neuroangiogenesis. Am J Pathol 188: 2281–2292, 2018. PMCID: 6169127)

randomized, placebo-controlled trials, medroxyprogesterone acetate, danazol, GnRHa, and the GnRH antagonist were all more effective than placebo. Pain relief of more than 6 months' duration was noted in 40–70% of women [53]. Although they are not formally FDA endorsed, continuous oral contraceptives also have been found to be efficacious and are widely used [54]. Following surgery for endometriomas, oral contraceptives significantly reduced pain and recurrence when compared to controls. Progestin-containing intrauterine systems have also shown merit to ameliorate post-operative endometriosis-induced dysmenorrhea.

Although highly effective in the management of pain with endometriosis, treatment with GnRHa or the oral antagonist is limited to 6 months by the FDA because of the risk of hypoestrogenic effects induced by ovarian suppression, including loss of bone mineral density. Suppression of the hypothalamic–pituitary axis by these agents can be mitigated with "add-back" of exogenous ovarian steroids. Add-back regimens with norethindrone acetate combined with low-dose estrogen can safely extend pain relief and bone preservation for at least 1 year, and one trial, with a limited number of participants, found no ill effects after 10 years of treatment with add-back therapy [55]. Randomized, clinical trials demonstrated that the 6 months of subcutaneous progestin was as effective as GnRHa in diminishing endometriosis-associated pain, but drop-out rates were significant for both treatment groups. Purported benefits of the progestin are ease of administration, decreased costs, and protection of bone mineral density. The role of the etonogestrel implant in this setting is addressed by Di Carlo in Chap. 7 of this text.

Dopamine receptor-2 agonists, with purported anti-angiogenic properties, have shown some promise in pre-clinical trials. Complementary and alternative medicine (CAM) in the form of medicinal herbs and isoflavones, which are plant-derived nonsteroidal substances, are claimed to have beneficial effects but require more rigorous human studies to further substantiate.

Different classes of immunomodulatory drugs are in stages of development that hold promise as future endometriosis therapeutics. Small molecule anti-rheumatic agents (e.g., hydroxychloroquine), c-Jun N-terminal kinase inhibitors (e.g., bentamapimod), statins (e.g., simvastatin), peroxisome proliferator activated receptor-$\gamma$ ligands (e.g., pioglitazone) and some biologics (e.g., infliximab, interferon-$\alpha$) have shown salutary effects in cellular and animal models, although few have been studied in clinical trials [56]. In addition to these, several repurposed medications have been shown in preclinical studies to have activities that are useful for the suppression of inflammation and pain. For example, bortezomib (a proteasome inhibitor that targets multiple myeloma), digitoxin (the cardiac glycoside), and tioconazole (an imidazole antifungal) are all FDA-approved drugs with proven in vitro NF-$\kappa$B inhibitor activity [57]. This topic is comprehensively reviewed in the accompanying Chap. 5 by Petraglia and colleagues.

## 4.6    Conclusions

Endometriosis-associated pelvic pain has been recognized for centuries, but its etiology and pathogenesis remain topics of continued debate and investigation. Based on the classical theory first promoted by Sampson, we offer a step-wise hypothesis that explains how interactions of the endocrine and immune systems affect nascent endometriosis lesions (Fig. 4.1). Each of the multiple nodes in this cascade is potential target for new endometriosis treatment strategies. As reviewed in this monograph by Professor Nisolle (Chap. 9), more and more refined surgical methods continue to play a major role in the management of pelvic pain associated with endometriosis. As our knowledge of pain pathophysiology evolves we expect that many, less invasive alternatives can be developed and introduced to clinical care.

# References

1. Laghzaoui O, Laghzaoui M. Nasal endometriosis: apropos of 1 case. J Gynecol Obstet Biol Reprod (Paris). 2001;30:786–8.
2. Buck Louis GM, Hediger ML, Peterson CM, Croughan M, Sundaram R, Stanford J, Chen Z, Fujimoto VY, Varner MW, Trumble A, Giudice LC. Incidence of endometriosis by study population and diagnostic method: the ENDO study. Fertil Steril. 2011;96:360–5.
3. Taylor HS, Giudice LC, Lessey BA, Abrao MS, Kotarski J, Archer DF, Diamond MP, Surrey E, Johnson NP, Watts NB, Gallagher JC, Simon JA, Carr BR, Dmowski WP, Leyland N, Rowan JP, Duan WR, Ng J, Schwefel B, Thomas JW, Jain RI, Chwalisz K. Treatment of endometriosis-associated pain with elagolix, an oral GnRH antagonist. N Engl J Med. 2017;377:28–40.
4. Anaf V, Simon P, El Nakadi I, Fayt I, Simonart T, Buxant F, Noel JC. Hyperalgesia, nerve infiltration and nerve growth factor expression in deep adenomyotic nodules, peritoneal and ovarian endometriosis. Hum Reprod. 2002;17:1895–900.
5. Evans S, Moalem-Taylor G, Tracey DJ. Pain and endometriosis. Pain. 2007;132(Suppl 1): S22–5.
6. Asante A, Taylor RN. Endometriosis: the role of neuroangiogenesis. Annu Rev Physiol. 2011;73:163–82.
7. As-Sanie S, Kim J, Schmidt-Wilcke T, Sundgren PC, Clauw DJ, Napadow V, Harris RE. Functional connectivity is associated with altered brain chemistry in women with endometriosis-associated chronic pelvic pain. J Pain. 2016;17:1–13.
8. Treloar SA, O'Connor DT, O'Connor VM, Martin NG. Genetic influences on endometriosis in an Australian twin sample. Fertil Steril. 1999;71:701–10.
9. Zondervan KT, Becker CM, Koga K, Missmer SA, Taylor RN, Vigano P. Endometriosis. Nat Rev Dis Primers. 2018;4:9.
10. Simpson JL, Elias S, Malinak LR, Buttram VC Jr. Heritable aspects of endometriosis. I. Genetic studies. Am J Obstet Gynecol. 1980;137:327–31.
11. Knapp VJ. How old is endometriosis? Late 17th- and 18th-century European descriptions of the disease. Fertil Steril. 1999;72:10–4.
12. Sampson JA. Peritoneal endometriosis due to menstrual dissemination of endometrial tissue into the peritoneal cavity. Am J Obstet Gynecol. 1927;14:442–69.
13. Halme J, Hammond MG, Hulka JF, Raj SG, Talbert LM. Retrograde menstruation in healthy women and in patients with endometriosis. Obstet Gynecol. 1984;64:151–4.
14. Stuparich MA, Donnellan NM, Sanfilippo JS. Endometriosis in the adolescent patient. Semin Reprod Med. 2017;35:102–9.
15. Vercellini P, Pisacreta A, Pesole A, Vicentini S, Stellato G, Crosignani PG. Is ureteral endometriosis an asymmetric disease? BJOG. 2000;107:559–61.
16. Jiang QY, Wu RJ. Growth mechanisms of endometriotic cells in implanted places: a review. Gynecol Endocrinol. 2012;28:562–7.
17. Laschke MW, Menger MD. Basic mechanisms of vascularization in endometriosis and their clinical implications. Hum Reprod Update. 2018;24(2):207–24.
18. Mueller MD, Vigne JL, Minchenko A, Lebovic DI, Leitman DC, Taylor RN. Regulation of vascular endothelial growth factor (VEGF) gene transcription by estrogen receptors alpha and beta. Proc Natl Acad Sci U S A. 2000;97:10972–7.
19. Barbieri RL. Endometriosis and the estrogen threshold theory. Relation to surgical and medical treatment. J Reprod Med. 1998;43:287–92.
20. Riggs MM, Bennetts M, van der Graaf PH, Martin SW. Integrated pharmacometrics and systems pharmacology model-based analyses to guide GnRH receptor modulator development for management of endometriosis. CPT Pharmacometrics Syst Pharmacol. 2012;1:e11. https://doi.org/10.1038/psp.2012.10.:e11.

21. Vitonis AF, Baer HJ, Hankinson SE, Laufer MR, Missmer SA. A prospective study of body size during childhood and early adulthood and the incidence of endometriosis. Hum Reprod. 2010;25:1325–34.
22. Yilmaz BD, Bulun SE. Endometriosis and nuclear receptors. Hum Reprod Update. 2019;25:473–85.
23. Reis FM, Petraglia F, Taylor RN. Endometriosis: hormone regulation and clinical consequences of chemotaxis and apoptosis. Hum Reprod Update. 2013;19:406–18.
24. Xue Q, Lin Z, Cheng YH, Huang CC, Marsh E, Yin P, Milad MP, Confino E, Reierstad S, Innes J, Bulun SE. Promoter methylation regulates estrogen receptor 2 in human endometrium and endometriosis. Biol Reprod. 2007;77:681–7.
25. Struller F, Weinreich FJ, Horvath P, Kokkalis MK, Beckert S, Konigsrainer A, Reymond MA. Peritoneal innervation: embryology and functional anatomy. Pleura Peritoneum. 2017;2:153–61.
26. Anaf V, Simon P, El Nakadi I, Fayt I, Buxant F, Simonart T, Peny MO, Noel JC. Relationship between endometriotic foci and nerves in rectovaginal endometriotic nodules. Hum Reprod. 2000;15:1744–50.
27. Tulandi T, Felemban A, Chen MF. Nerve fibers and histopathology of endometriosis-harboring peritoneum. J Am Assoc Gynecol Laparosc. 2001;8:95–8.
28. Berkley KJ, Dmitrieva N, Curtis KS, Papka RE. Innervation of ectopic endometrium in a rat model of endometriosis. Proc Natl Acad Sci U S A. 2004;101:11094–8.
29. Tokushige N, Markham R, Russell P, Fraser IS. Nerve fibres in peritoneal endometriosis. Hum Reprod. 2006;21:3001–7.
30. Tokushige N, Markham R, Russell P, Fraser IS. High density of small nerve fibres in the functional layer of the endometrium in women with endometriosis. Hum Reprod. 2006;21:782–7.
31. Bokor A, Kyama CM, Vercruysse L, Fassbender A, Gevaert O, Vodolazkaia A, De Moor B, Fulop V, D'Hooghe T. Density of small diameter sensory nerve fibres in endometrium: a semi-invasive diagnostic test for minimal to mild endometriosis. Hum Reprod. 2009;24:3025–32.
32. Borghese B, Vaiman D, Mondon F, Mbaye M, Anaf V, Noel JC, de Ziegler D, Chapron C. Neurotrophins and pain in endometriosis. Gynecol Obstet Fertil. 2010;38:442–6.
33. Kajitani T, Maruyama T, Asada H, Uchida H, Oda H, Uchida S, Miyazaki K, Arase T, Ono M, Yoshimura Y. Possible involvement of nerve growth factor in dysmenorrhea and dyspareunia associated with endometriosis. Endocr J. 2013;60:1155–64.
34. Garcia-Solares J, Dolmans MM, Squifflet JL, Donnez J, Donnez O. Invasion of human deep nodular endometriotic lesions is associated with collective cell migration and nerve development. Fertil Steril. 2018;110:1318–27.
35. Williams C, Hoang L, Yosef A, Alotaibi F, Allaire C, Brotto L, Fraser IS, Bedaiwy MA, Ng TL, Lee AF, Yong PJ. Nerve bundles and deep dyspareunia in endometriosis. Reprod Sci. 2016;23:892–901.
36. Browne AS, Yu J, Huang RP, Francisco AM, Sidell N, Taylor RN. Proteomic identification of neurotrophins in the eutopic endometrium of women with endometriosis. Fertil Steril. 2012;98:713–9.
37. Rocha AL, Vieira EL, Ferreira MC, Maia LM, Teixeira AL, Reis FM. Plasma brain-derived neurotrophic factor in women with pelvic pain: a potential biomarker for endometriosis? Biomark Med. 2017;11:313–7.
38. Nisenblat V, Bossuyt PM, Shaikh R, Farquhar C, Jordan V, Scheffers CS, Mol BW, Johnson N, Hull ML. Blood biomarkers for the non-invasive diagnosis of endometriosis. Cochrane Database Syst Rev. 2016:CD012179.
39. Shifren JL, Tseng JF, Zaloudek CJ, Ryan IP, Meng YG, Ferrara N, Jaffe RB, Taylor RN. Ovarian steroid regulation of vascular endothelial growth factor in the human endometrium: implications for angiogenesis during the menstrual cycle and in the pathogenesis of endometriosis. J Clin Endocrinol Metab. 1996;81:3112–8.

40. Donnez J, Smoes P, Gillerot S, Casanas-Roux F, Nisolle M. Vascular endothelial growth factor (VEGF) in endometriosis. Hum Reprod. 1998;13:1686–90.
41. Carmeliet P, Tessier-Lavigne M. Common mechanisms of nerve and blood vessel wiring. Nature. 2005;436:193–200.
42. Raab S, Plate KH. Different networks, common growth factors: shared growth factors and receptors of the vascular and the nervous system. Acta Neuropathol. 2007;113:607–26.
43. Asally R, Markham R, Manconi F. The expression and cellular localisation of Neurotrophin and neural guidance molecules in peritoneal ectopic lesions. Mol Neurobiol. 2019;56:4013–22.
44. McKinnon B, Bersinger NA, Wotzkow C, Mueller MD. Endometriosis-associated nerve fibers, peritoneal fluid cytokine concentrations, and pain in endometriotic lesions from different locations. Fertil Steril. 2012;97:373–80.
45. Liang Y, Liu D, Yang F, Pan W, Zeng F, Wu J, Xie H, Li J, Yao S. Perineural invasion in endometriotic lesions contributes to endometriosis-associated pain. J Pain Res. 2018;11:1999–2009.
46. Harp D, Driss A, Mehrabi S, Chowdhury I, Xu W, Liu D, Garcia-Barrio M, Taylor RN, Gold B, Jefferson S, Sidell N, Thompson W. Exosomes derived from endometriotic stromal cells have enhanced angiogenic effects in vitro. Cell Tissue Res. 2016;365:187–96.
47. Sun H, Li D, Yuan M, Li Q, Li N, Wang G. Eutopic stromal cells of endometriosis promote neuroangiogenesis via exosome pathwaydagger. Biol Reprod. 2019;100:649–59.
48. Wessels JM, Leyland NA, Agarwal SK, Foster WG. Estrogen induced changes in uterine brain-derived neurotrophic factor and its receptors. Hum Reprod. 2015;30:925–36.
49. Yu J, Francisco AMC, Patel BG, Cline JM, Zou E, Berga SL, Taylor RN. IL-1beta stimulates brain-derived neurotrophic factor production in Eutopic endometriosis stromal cell cultures: a model for cytokine regulation of neuroangiogenesis. Am J Pathol. 2018;188:2281–92.
50. Forster R, Sarginson A, Velichkova A, Hogg C, Dorning A, Horne AW, Saunders PTK, Greaves E. Macrophage-derived insulin-like growth factor-1 is a key neurotrophic and nerve-sensitizing factor in pain associated with endometriosis. FASEB J. 2019;33:11210–22.
51. As-Sanie S, Harris RE, Napadow V, Kim J, Neshewat G, Kairys A, Williams D, Clauw DJ, Schmidt-Wilcke T. Changes in regional gray matter volume in women with chronic pelvic pain: a voxel-based morphometry study. Pain. 2012;153:1006–14.
52. Coxon L, Horne AW, Vincent K. Pathophysiology of endometriosis-associated pain: a review of pelvic and central nervous system mechanisms. Best Pract Res Clin Obstet Gynaecol. 2018;51:53–67.
53. Howard FM. An evidence-based medicine approach to the treatment of endometriosis-associated chronic pelvic pain: placebo-controlled studies. J Am Assoc Gynecol Laparosc. 2000;7:477–88.
54. Vercellini P, Frontino G, De GO, Pietropaolo G, Pasin R, Crosignani PG. Continuous use of an oral contraceptive for endometriosis-associated recurrent dysmenorrhea that does not respond to a cyclic pill regimen. Fertil Steril. 2003;80:560–3.
55. Surrey ES, Hornstein MD. Prolonged GnRH agonist and add-back therapy for symptomatic endometriosis: long-term follow-up. Obstet Gynecol. 2002;99:709–19.
56. Kotlyar A, Taylor HS, D'Hooghe TM. Use of immunomodulators to treat endometriosis. Best Pract Res Clin Obstet Gynaecol. 2019;60:56–65.
57. Miller SC, Huang R, Sakamuru S, Shukla SJ, Attene-Ramos MS, Shinn P, Van Leer D, Leister W, Austin CP, Xia M. Identification of known drugs that act as inhibitors of NF-kappaB signaling and their mechanism of action. Biochem Pharmacol. 2010;79:1272–80.

# Endometriosis-Induced Pain: The Treatment Strategy

# 5

Sara Clemenza, Tommaso Capezzuoli, Huixi Chen, Massimiliano Fambrini, and Felice Petraglia

## 5.1 Introduction

Pain is one of the main symptoms in women with endometriosis. Dysmenorrhea, chronic pelvic pain (CPP), dyspareunia, back pain, and dyschezia are the most common pain manifestations [1]. No relationship between endometriosis stage and painful symptoms (presence and severity) is present. The mechanism of endometriosis-associated pain remains unclear but multiple factors are involved, like nociception, inflammation, and alterations in peripheral and central nervous system pain processing [2, 3]. In addition, psychological aspects also play a role in pain development [4].

S. Clemenza · T. Capezzuoli · M. Fambrini
Division of Obstetrics and Gynecology, Department of Biomedical, Experimental and Clinical Sciences "Mario Serio", University of Florence, Florence, Italy

H. Chen
Division of Obstetrics and Gynecology, Department of Biomedical, Experimental and Clinical Sciences "Mario Serio", University of Florence, Florence, Italy

International Peace Maternity and Child Health Hospital, School of Medicine, Shanghai Jiao Tong University, Shangai, China

F. Petraglia (✉)
Obstetrics and Gynecology Division, University of Florence, Florence, Italy
e-mail: felice.petraglia@unifi.it

© International Society of Gynecological Endocrinology 2021
A. R. Genazzani et al. (eds.), *Endometriosis Pathogenesis, Clinical Impact and Management*, ISGE Series, https://doi.org/10.1007/978-3-030-57866-4_5

## 5.2    Pathogenesis of Endometriosis-Associated Pain

### 5.2.1    Peripheral Pain Mechanisms

A typical endometriosis feature is hyperalgesia, an abnormally high sensation of pain when a not painful stimulus is applied. Hyperalgesia is a characteristic of neuropathic pain, usually related to nerve injury or inflammatory stimulus.

The local nerve fibers activated by increased inflammatory and neurogenic factors and the direct infiltration of the peripheral nerves by endometriotic stromal cells may contribute to this phenomenon [3].

Perineural and intraneural invasion of endometriotic glands or stromal cells were found in deep endometriosis lesions [5]. Moreover, immune mediators (cytokines, interleukins, growth factors) are upregulated in the peritoneal fluid of women with endometriosis. Histamine, tryptase, serotonin, monocyte chemotactic protein-1 (MCP-1), tumor necrosis factors (TNF), interleukins (IL)-1, -6, and -8, prostaglandins and nerve growth factors (NGF) are abnormally synthesized and released by activated macrophages, mast cells, NK cells and leukocytes within the endometriotic lesions, close to sensory nerve fibers, and in the peritoneal fluid [2, 6, 7]. Inflammatory molecules sensitize (lower the threshold) or excite the terminals of sensory nerve fibers, causing the development of a vicious cycle characterized by nociceptor sensitization, local neo-neurogenesis, and activation of sensory nerve fibers, leading to hyperalgesia [2, 7].

### 5.2.2    Central Pain Mechanisms

Nociceptor inputs can trigger a phenomenon called "central sensitization" that represents an enhancement in the function of neurons and circuits in nociceptive pathways caused by increases in membrane excitability and synaptic efficacy [8]. It might play a role in CPP [9] and in endometriosis-associated pain [10].

Changes in structure and function of Central Nervous System (CNS) in women with endometriosis-associated pain have been shown: in particular, they showed lower gray matter (GM) volume in brain regions involved in pain transmission (left thalamus, left cingulate gyrus, right putamen, and right insula) and larger GM volume in regions involved in pain modulation and endocrine function regulation [11]. These data suggest that the presence of a central pain in endometriosis is reflected by changes in regional brain morphology [12]. Supporting this concept, women with endometriosis-related CPP show a higher concentration of excitatory neurotransmitters in the anterior insula and a greater intrinsic connectivity between the same cerebral region and the medial prefrontal cortex [13], suggesting a central sensitization in women with endometriosis. Similar morphological brain changes have been observed in other recurrent or chronic pain states, while these changes were not observed in patients with endometriosis who had no CPP.

The involvement of the hypothalamic–pituitary–adrenal axis (HPA) in women with endometriosis is also supposed by reduced salivary cortisol levels [14, 15].

While acute stress leads to the activation of the HPA axis and an increase in cortisol levels, chronic pain attenuates this response. In fact, this may be beneficial for an individual, as continued activation of the body's 'emergency response' systems could lead to further tissue damage both locally and systemically. However, low levels of cortisol may exacerbate painful symptoms by reducing the endogenous analgesia associated with stress, that is thought to facilitate the 'fight-flight response'. Central changes in women with endometriosis may explain why therapies directed at the periphery fail to relieve pain, and pain becomes increasingly difficult to treat. Additionally, it is plausible that these central changes contribute to the disparity between the extent of disease observed at laparoscopy and the pain experienced [16].

### 5.2.3  Other Pain Mechanisms

Pain experience may cause psychological and cognitive disorders including depression, anxiety, and belief states [4, 9, 10]. The balance between peripheral and central influences and identifying eventual emotional or cognitive disorders may be helpful in the planning of a correct and individualized treatment.

Finally, the complications of previous surgical procedures for endometriosis could be a possible pathogenetic factor of pain [9]. The main complications following surgery of endometriosis are infection, vaginal vault hematoma, pelvic hemorrhage, autonomic nerve injury, adhesion, and fistula formation, which may also contribute to pain symptoms [17].

The pathogenetic mechanisms underlie endometriosis-associated pain are summarized in Fig. 5.1.

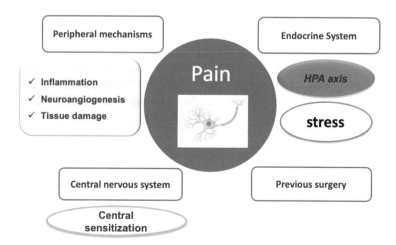

**Fig. 5.1**  Pain mechanisms in endometriosis

## 5.3    Different Diagnosis of Pelvic Pain

Endometriosis symptoms, especially chronic pelvic pain, are similar to those found in other gynecological and non-gynecological conditions. Adenomyosis, pelvic adhesions, pelvic inflammatory disease, congenital anomalies of the reproductive tract, and ovarian or tubal masses can cause chronic pelvic pain. Moreover, gastro-intestinal, urinary, neurologic, musculoskeletal, and psychiatric disorders can be associated with pelvic pain. Therefore, a careful evaluation to exclude other causes of pelvic pain should be pursued before aggressive therapy and also in those women who do not respond to conventional therapy for endometriosis [18]. Finally, the presence of associated uterine disorders (adenomyosis and uterine myomas), systemic and psychiatric comorbidities should be carefully evaluated [19, 20].

## 5.4    Treatment of Endometriosis-Associated Pain

The management of women with endometriosis-associated pelvic pain is both medical and surgical. Patients have to be counseled that no treatment is curative since the disease is chronic, progressive, and tends to recur after stopping any treatment. Since endometriosis affects women between 16 and 45 years and has different phenotypes, the therapeutic choice should take into account the characteristics of each individual patient, age, and the desire of pregnancy, as well as the phenotype. Endometriosis constitutes a paradigm for the new model of patient-centered medicine: a wide variety of treatments targeting different pathways are important to develop a personalized medicine in endometriosis [21].

The therapeutic choices for the treatment of endometriosis-associated pain are summarized in Fig. 5.2.

### 5.4.1    Medical Therapy

Medical therapy should be conceived as a long-term treatment, similar to therapy for other chronic inflammatory conditions. The objectives of medical management include relief of pain, prevention of recurrence, and enhancing fertility in women who desire to have children.

They are classified into hormonal and non-hormonal treatments. Currently, first-line hormonal drugs act by blocking ovarian function, thereby creating a state of iatrogenic menopause or pseudopregnancy. The common medical treatments create a hypoestrogenic environment either by blocking ovarian estrogen secretion or by inhibiting estrogenic stimulation of the ectopic endometrium [18]. Therefore, the main limitation of current hormonal treatments is the antiovulatory effect for women seeking pregnancy.

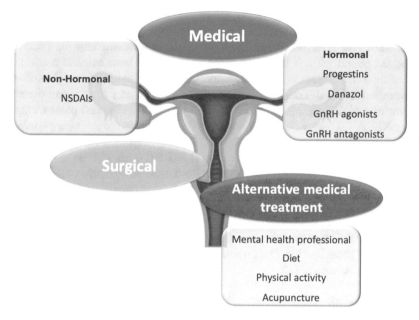

**Fig. 5.2** Treatment of endometriosis-associated pain

### 5.4.1.1 Nonsteroidal Anti-Inflammatory Drugs (NSDAIs)

NSDAIs interfere with the function of the enzyme COX-1 and COX-2, inhibiting the conversion of arachidonic acid to prostaglandins, involved in the genesis of endometriosis-associated pain. NSAIDs provide effective treatment for women with pain caused by primary dysmenorrhoea and appear to be the only medical option consistent with the maintenance of fertility. However, women using NSAIDs are aware that these drugs may cause unintended effects, especially in gastrointestinal, cardiovascular, and nervous system [22].

### 5.4.1.2 Progestins

The progestins should be considered as the first-choice treatment in the presence of painful symptoms. Progestins induce atrophy of eutopic and ectopic endometrium and have anti-inflammatory and pro-apoptotic properties. Moreover, they induce suppression of matrix metalloproteinases, a class of enzymes important in the growth and implantation of ectopic endometrium. Their use is associated with the improvement of pain and quality of life in two-thirds of patients. Progestins can be administered by oral, intramuscular, subcutaneous, and intrauterine route.

Norethisterone acetate (NETA) and dienogest, 19-nortestosterone derivatives, are the most used progestins (at the dose of 2.5–5.0 mg/day and 2 mg/day, respectively). NETA has stronger progestogenic effects than dienogest, but it also has androgenic activity, whereas dienogest is antiandrogenic. Oral NETA is particularly effective in patients with deep dyspareunia and rectovaginal lesions with gradual but progressive pain reduction during the time. Some side effects of NETA are caused by the residual androgenic activity (weight gain, acne, and seborrhea). NETA is partly metabolized to estradiol and does not cause hypoestrogenic effects and may be used for a prolonged period without detrimental consequences on bone mineral content. The use of oral dienogest is supported by the largest evidence originated from Randomized Clinical Trials and cohort studies. It is better than placebo and not inferior to a GnRH agonist in relieving endometriosis-associated pain. Compared with NETA it was similarly effective on pain but better tolerated [23, 24]. Medroxyprogesterone acetate (DMPA) may constitute an alternative treatment. Levonorgestrel-intrauterine device (LNG-IUD) should be considered in women who do not tolerate progestins. LNG-IUD is particularly useful in parous women with no further pregnancy desire and with dysmenorrhea as the main symptom [23, 24]. Progestins are safe and very effective in women with deep infiltrating endometriosis with severe dyspareunia, including those patients with bowel nodules. The most common side effect of progestins is irregular bleeding. In the case of persistent bleeding, discontinuing treatment for some days is effective in restoring amenorrhea [23].

### 5.4.1.3 Danazol

Danazol, a derivative of 17α-ethynyl testosterone, induces the inhibition of gonadotropin release and has a strong anti-estrogenic activity. It is effective at treating endometriosis-related pain, but its use is limited by the androgenic-type adverse effects such as seborrhea, hypertrichosis, weight gain, HDL levels reduction, and LDL levels increase. Good efficacy and tolerability are reported with vaginal use of danazol (200 mg/day) [25, 26].

### 5.4.1.4 Gonadotropin-Releasing Hormone (GnRH) Agonists

GnRH agonists (Leuprolide and Triptorelin) are effective in the relief of pain. These compounds bind to the pituitary GnRH receptors and, after an initial stimulation of pituitary release of LH and FSH, a downregulation of the pituitary–ovarian axis and hypoestrogenism occurs. The hypoestrogenic state is responsible for significant side effects, including hot flushes, vaginal dryness, and osteopenia. The addition of estro-progestins add-back therapy reduces these adverse effects, without reducing the efficacy of pain relief. GnRH agonists are approved for only up to 6 months of continuous use, but the add-back therapy can permit longer-term use [27].

### 5.4.1.5 GnRH Antagonist

The main advantage of GnRH antagonists is the immediate blockage of the GnRH receptor, without the initial stimulation of the hypothalamic–pituitary–gonadal axis (flare up). The "estrogen threshold hypothesis" was the hypothesis that could favor the use of GnRH antagonists holding the amount of estrogen, necessary to prevent hot flushes, bone loss, and other hypoestrogenic symptoms and side effects. Elagolix, a short-acting, oral, non-peptide GnRH antagonist, has been recently approved in the United States for the management of moderate to severe pain associated with endometriosis (150 mg once daily or 200 mg twice daily). Higher doses of Elagolix are the most effective in reducing pain but are more frequently associated with the side effects of hypoestrogenism (hot flash, decrease in bone mineral density and increase in serum lipid levels). Currently, ongoing trials are evaluating the safety and efficacy of Elagolix with an add-back therapy [22].

### 5.4.1.6 Other Medical Treatment Under Investigation

Medical treatment options for endometriosis currently under investigation include Selective estrogen receptor modulators (SERM), Selective progesterone receptor modulators (SPRM), immunomodulatory drugs, statins, antiangiogenic agents, Histone deacetylase inhibitor, Icon, Peroxisome proliferator receptor g (PPARg), dopaminergic agonists, and cannabinoids. Aromatase inhibitors (AIs) block estrogen synthesis both in the periphery and in the ovaries causing hypoestrogenism; therefore, their use should be associated with add-back therapy. AIs should be used off-label especially in women with severe pain refractory to other medical or surgical treatments [22, 27]. However, most of the studies conducted are experimental and proved to be efficacious in animal studies. Thus, further studies are necessary to support their introduction into routine clinical practice [22].

## 5.5 Surgical Treatments

Laparoscopic surgical removal of endometriosis is an effective approach for the treatment of pain associated with endometriosis. However, because of the complexity of the interventions, the average young age of patients, the possible desire for offspring, and the high rate of recurrence, surgery has limited indications and should be proposed as a second line after medical therapy.

Surgery is indicated for symptomatic or large endometriomas. Ovarian cystectomy is the more effective procedure for improving symptoms of dysmenorrhea, dyspareunia, non-menstrual pelvic pain, and recurrence of the endometrioma compared to drainage and electrocoagulation. However, women with endometrioma should be informed that surgery potentially reduces ovarian reserve. A correct surgical procedure reduces damage to the residual ovarian tissue and increases the chances of pregnancy.

Surgery for deep infiltrating endometriosis is effective, but it is associated with significant complication rates. Therefore, surgical treatment for pelvic endometriosis should be reserved for superficial or infiltrating forms of endometriosis not responsive to drug treatment or with contraindications to hormonal medical therapy. Moreover, repeated surgery should be avoided, because of the possible formation of abdominal–pelvic adhesions, which can worsen painful symptoms.

The surgeon should have experience also in extragenital problems, such as urological or colorectal surgical procedures ("pelvic surgeon"). In some cases, the treatment should be carried out by a multidisciplinary team that includes the gynecologist, general surgeon, and urologist. A possible option in the treatment of deep endometriosis is neuro ablation, in particular uterine nerve ablation (UNA) and presacral neurectomy (PSN) [18].

## 5.6    Alternative Pain Treatments

Endometriosis may be associated with severe psychosocial consequences such as anxiety, depression, isolation, familial and intimate implications including unfavorable emotional impact in partners, decreased quality of life, inability to cope with everyday activities, reduced work productivity, and greatly increased expenditure on health care. Therefore, a mental health professional should be considered to address the psychological stress and depression that may be associated with chronic pelvic pain. It can also be helpful to involve a pain management specialist to coordinate analgesic treatment as well as to provide other modalities such as neuroleptic drugs and nerve blocks [4].

Diet, dietary supplements, and herbal medicine are often proposed and/or used as adjuncts without any conclusive evidence. Moreover, physical adjunctive therapies such as acupuncture, transcutaneous neurostimulation, osteopathy/chiropractic, and physical activity may potentiate beneficial effects perceived by patients. However, it remains difficult to demonstrate significant effects of cognitive and/or behavioral interventions on endometriosis-related pain [28].

## 5.7    Conclusion

Endometriosis is characterized by multiple clinical phenotypes and multiform symptomatology. Nevertheless, pelvic pain is almost constantly present and represents one of the most important characteristics of the disorders. Progestins are the first-choice medical treatment in endometriosis patients and are particularly effective in case of deep infiltrating endometriosis, with or without severe dyspareunia. Surgery is useful in selected cases but it is characterized by several limitations, such as the presence of complications and the negative effect on the ovarian reserve. Compared to the past, the management of endometriosis is mainly based on the use of medical treatments, avoiding repeated surgical procedures. Endometriosis management should be individualized and patient-oriented and not standardized.

## References

1. Vercellini P, Vigano P, Somigliana E, Fedele L. Endometriosis: pathogenesis and treatment. Nat Rev Endocrinol. 2014;10:261–75.
2. Howard FM. Endometriosis and mechanisms of pelvic pain. J Minim Invasive Gynecol. 2009;16:540–50.
3. Morotti M, Vincent K, Becker CM. Mechanisms of pain in endometriosis. Eur J Obstet Gynecol Reprod Biol. 2017;209:8–13.
4. Vannuccini S, Reis FM, Coutinho LM, Lazzeri L, Centini G, Petraglia F. Surgical treatment of endometriosis: prognostic factors for better quality of life. Gynecol Endocrinol. 2019;35 (11):1010–4.
5. Anaf V, Simon P, El Nakadi I, Fayt I, Buxant F, Simonart T, Peny MO, Noel JC. Relationship between endometriotic foci and nerves in rectovaginal endometriotic nodules. Hum Reprod. 2000;15:1744–50.

6. Gori M, Luddi A, Belmonte G, Piomboni P, Tosti C, Funghi L, Zupi E, Lazzeri L, Petraglia F. Expression of microtubule associated protein 2 and synaptophysin in endometrium: high levels in deep infiltrating endometriosis lesions. Fertil Steril. 2016;105(2):435–43.
7. Riccio L, Santulli P, Marcellin L, Abrao MS, Batteux F, Chapron C. Immunology of endometriosis. Best Pract Res Clin Obstet Gynaecol. 2018;50:39–49.
8. Woolf CJ. Central sensitization: implications for the diagnosis and treatment of pain. Pain. 2011;152:S2–15.
9. Brawn J, Morotti M, Zondervan KT, Becker CM, Vincent K. Central changes associated with chronic pelvic pain and endometriosis. Hum Reprod Update. 2014;20:737–47.
10. Vitonis AF, Vincent K, Rahmioglu N, Fassbender A, Buck Louis GM, Hummelshoj L, Giudice LC, Stratton P, Adamson GD, Becker CM, Zondervan KT, Missmer SA, WERF EPHect Working Group. World endometriosis research foundation endometriosis phenome and biobanking harmonization project: ii. Clinical and covariate phenotype data collection in endometriosis research. Fertil Steril. 2014;102:1223–32.
11. As-Sanie S, Harris RE, Napadow V, Kim J, Neshewat G, Kairys A, Williams D, Clauw DJ, Schmidt-Wilcke T. Changes in regional gray matter volume in women with chronic pelvic pain: a voxel-based morphometry study. Pain. 2012;153:1006–14.
12. Eippert F, Tracey I. Pain and the Pag: learning from painful mistakes. Nat Neurosci. 2014;17:1438–9.
13. As-Sanie S, Kim J, Schmidt-Wilcke T, Sundgren PC, Clauw DJ, Napadow V, Harris RE. Functional connectivity is associated with altered brain chemistry in women with endometriosis-associated chronic pelvic pain. J Pain. 2016;17:1–13.
14. Quiñones M, Urrutia R, Torres-Reverón A, Vincent K, Flores I. Anxiety, coping skills and hypothalamus-pituitary-adrenal (HPA) axis in patients with endometriosis. J Reprod Biol Health. 2015;3:pii: 2.
15. Petrelluzzi KF, Garcia MC, Petta CA, Grassi-Kassisse DM, Spadari-Bratfisch RC. Salivary cortisol concentrations, stress and quality of life in women with endometriosis and chronic pelvic pain. Stress. 2008;11:390–7.
16. Coxon L, Horne AW, Vincent K. Pathophysiology of endometriosis-associated pain: a review of pelvic and central nervous system mechanisms. Best Pract Res Clin Obstet Gynaecol. 2018;51:53–67. https://doi.org/10.1016/j.bpobgyn.2018.01.014
17. Guerra A, Daraï E, Osório F, Setúbal A, Bendifallah S, Loureiro A, Thomassin-Naggara I. Imaging of postoperative endometriosis. Diagn Interv Imaging. 2019;100:607–18.
18. Practice Committee of the American Society for Reproductive Medicine. Treatment of pelvic pain associated with endometriosis: a committee opinion. Fertil Steril. 2014;101:927–35.
19. Choi EJ, Cho SB, Lee SR, Lim YM, Jeong K, Moon HS, Chung H. Comorbidity of gynecological and non-gynecological diseases with adenomyosis and endometriosis. Obstet Gynecol Sci. 2017;60(6):579–86.
20. Vannuccini S, Lazzeri L, Orlandini C, Morgante G, Bifulco G, Fagiolini A, Petraglia F. Mental health, pain symptoms and systemic comorbidities in women with endometriosis: a cross-sectional study. J Psychosom Obstet Gynaecol. 2018;39(4):315–20.
21. Chapron C, Marcellin L, Borghese B, Santulli P. Rethinking mechanisms, diagnosis and management of endometriosis. Nat Rev Endocrinol. 2019;15(11):666–82.
22. Clemenza S, Sorbi F, Noci I, Capezzuoli T, Turrini I, Carriero C, Buffi N, Fambrini M, Petraglia F. From pathogenesis to clinical practice: emerging medical treatments for endometriosis. Best Pract Res Clin Obstet Gynaecol. 2018;51:92–101.
23. Vercellini P, Buggio L, Frattaruolo MP, Borghi A, Dridi D, Somigliana E. Medical treatment of endometriosis-related pain. Best Pract Res Clin Obstet Gynaecol. 2018;51:68–91.
24. Vercellini P, Buggio L, Berlanda N, Barbara G, Somigliana E, Bosari S. Estrogen-progestins and progestins for the management of endometriosis. Fertil Steril. 2016;106(7):1552–71.
25. Razzi S, Luisi S, Calonaci F, Altomare A, Bocchi C, Petraglia F. Efficacy of vaginal danazol treatment in women with recurrent deeply infiltrating endometriosis. Fertil Steril. 2007;88(4):789–94.

26. Tosti C, Pinzauti S, Santulli P, Chapron C, Petraglia F. Pathogenetic mechanisms of deep infiltrating endometriosis. Reprod Sci. 2015;22(9):1053–9.
27. Tosti C, Biscione A, Morgante G, Bifulco G, Luisi S, Petraglia F. Hormonal therapy for endometriosis: from molecular research to bedside. Eur J Obstet Gynecol Reprod Biol. 2017;209:61–6.
28. Wattier JM. Conventional analgesics and non-pharmacological multidisciplinary therapeutic treatment in endometriosis: CNGOF-HAS endometriosis guidelines. Gynecol Obstet Fertil Senol. 2018;46(3):248–55.

# Management of Endometriosis in Teenagers

**6**

Libera Troìa, Antonella Biscione, Irene Colombi, and Stefano Luisi

## 6.1 Introduction

Endometriosis in adolescents needs unique considerations for treatment approaches, as it presents particular challenges in terms of diagnosis, variable presentation and symptoms, and choice of treatment [1]. Dysmenorrhea is the most common gynecologic issue among adolescents, occurring in 50–80% of these and causing limitation in sports and activities, poor academic performance, and long duration of resting (Fig. 6.1). In about 10% of adolescents with severe dysmenorrhea symptoms, pelvic abnormalities such as endometriosis or uterine anomalies may be found and the incidence of endometriosis has been reported between 45% and 70% in adolescents with chronic pelvic pain (CPP) [2].

About the correlation between endometriosis and chronic pelvic pain, evidence supports an increased awareness among adolescents and their health care providers about the need for early clinical diagnosis of endometriosis and timely treatment of severe dysmenorrhea/pelvic pain, usually with medical therapy as first line and surgery as second line if the pain is not responsive to medical therapy and complication such as torsion or breakage risk of endometrioma occur [1, 3].

The targets for analgesic treatment fall into the usual categories of prevention or limiting the disease: peripherally acting and centrally acting medications, psychological approaches, and non-invasive procedures such as focused ultrasound. For chronic pain, the target is to reset the brain state using one or a combination of approaches (Fig. 6.2). Once the disease is diagnosed and treated, these patients have favorable outcomes with hormonal and non-hormonal therapy [4]; however, for those who do undergo surgery, about 30% of women still report ongoing pelvic pain after surgery despite taking medications. For these reasons in endometriosis,

L. Troìa · A. Biscione · I. Colombi · S. Luisi (✉)
Obstetrics and Gynecology, Department of Molecular and Developmental Medicine, University of Siena, Siena, Italy
e-mail: stefano.luisi@unisi.it

© International Society of Gynecological Endocrinology 2021
A. R. Genazzani et al. (eds.), *Endometriosis Pathogenesis, Clinical Impact and Management*, ISGE Series, https://doi.org/10.1007/978-3-030-57866-4_6

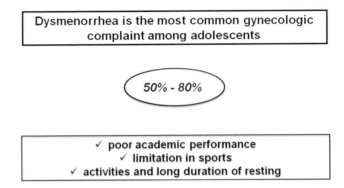

Dysmenorrhea is the most common gynecologic complaint among adolescents

50% - 80%

✓ poor academic performance
✓ limitation in sports
✓ activities and long duration of resting

**Fig. 6.1** The impact of dysmenorrhea in teenagers

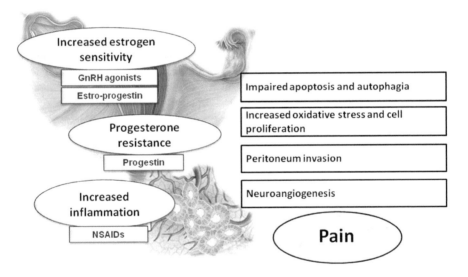

Increased estrogen sensitivity

GnRH agonists

Estro-progestin

Impaired apoptosis and autophagia

Increased oxidative stress and cell proliferation

Progesterone resistance

Progestin

Peritoneum invasion

Increased inflammation

Neuroangiogenesis

NSAIDs

Pain

**Fig. 6.2** The pathogenesis of endometriosis and its treatment options

multidimensional and personalized pain treatment has been difficult to achieve. There is a great need for a specific conceptual model for adolescents with endometriosis, in consideration that the younger the woman at onset of symptoms, the longer the duration until diagnosis is made [1].

## 6.1.1 Treatment Approaches

The World Endometriosis Society consensus states that early diagnosis and treatment—both medical and surgical modalities—have the potential of improving quality of life, alleviating symptoms, preventing the development of more severe disease later in life and minimizing the likelihood that future fertility may become compromised [5].

Although surgery is effective in treating endometriosis in adults, few studies have been conducted on adolescents and surgery should be carefully considered in these patients. Apart from the increased risk of premature ovarian failure caused by surgical treatment of ovarian endometriomas [6], recent animal and epidemiological studies indicate that surgery, in and by itself, may encourage the development of endometriosis [7]. In fact, a history of surgery for endometriosis is correlated with the presence and severity of deep infiltrating endometriosis, underlining the necessity of a thorough preoperative assessment and the need for providing comprehensive information to these patients before undertaking further surgery [8]. This is why medical treatments take special importance in treating adolescents. In principle, the same drugs can be used in adolescent and adult patients. The critical issue, however, is the progressive and dynamic nature of endometriosis, shown both in spontaneous and induced disease [9]. Once diagnosis is posed, no delay in treatment together with a combined medical–surgical approach, represent the key points to slow its progression. At any rate, an attempt with a medical regimen should be the first choice [10].

## 6.1.2  Medical Treatment

As there is a high prevalence of dysmenorrhea in adolescents, it is reasonable to empirically treat these patients with NSAIDs and/or COCPs, unless the patient has no contraindications to these therapies. The provider may choose to initiate at first COCPs cyclically. The duration of this initial treatment should generally be three menstrual cycles with close symptom follow-up to conclude if the patient has an appropriate response to therapy [11]. The use of a pain diary to assess possible changes in the pain is a good approach for this concern [12].

If this initial approach does not demonstrate adequate symptom improvement, then a change to continuous dosing of COCPs may be considered with the goal to induce amenorrhea and further diagnostic testing or examinations may also be considered. Indeed, it is important to remember that symptomatic improvement does not necessarily rule out endometriosis, so these patients must be counseled appropriately. Should the patient fail initial empiric therapy, it is important to maintain a high suspicion for a diagnosis of endometriosis.

It may be reasonable at this time to proceed with diagnostic laparoscopy and excision of endometriosis (if present), as 35–73% of these adolescents do have endometriosis at the time of surgery [11].

However, the provider should counsel the patient and her family on the role of attempting additional hormonal medical therapy with either progestin-only therapy or gonadotropin-releasing hormone (GnRH) agonists. These treatment modalities are options in patients who are not ideal candidates for surgical intervention or feel strongly about avoiding surgery altogether [11].

Because there is no surgical cure for endometriosis, all adolescents with endometriosis should be managed with long-term medical therapy to prevent the recurrence of symptoms and/or disease progression. An upstaging of disease at the time of second laparoscopy can occur if the patient was noncompliant with menstrual suppressive therapy [10].

Combination estrogen/progestin or progestin-only therapy serves to create a progestin-dominant environment, leading to decidualization and subsequent atrophy of intrauterine and extrauterine endometrial tissue [13].

There are no data suggesting that one pill formulation is better than another for the treatment of dysmenorrhea or endometriosis-associated pain. Thus, if one pill induces amenorrhea and pain persists, a different class of therapy should be considered. Alternatives for combined hormonal contraception include the vaginal ring or transdermal patch. All of these methods are safe and effective if given in a cyclic, extended, or continuous manner, but when treating endometriosis-associated pain, extended continuous use with menstrual suppression is recommended [13]. Progestin-only methods include the "mini-pill" (norethindrone only) or norethindrone acetate. It should be noted that there is a small peripheral conversion of norethindrone acetate to ethinyl estradiol, as opposed to norethindrone, which does not demonstrate conversion. Norethindrone acetate has been shown to be an effective treatment for endometriosis and tolerated by most adolescents [14]. Medroxyprogesterone acetate can also be used, and it is administered every 3 months in intramuscular or subcutaneous form. Progestin-only therapy has side effects that may not be well tolerated, such as irregular bleeding, acne, weight gain, and emotional lability. Providers should consider oral progestins prior to injectable therapy, to address side effects or to quickly discontinue the regimen. Depot medroxyprogesterone acetate (DMPA), in particular, can result in loss of bone density in some patients [4]. Alternative therapies include the etonogestrel implant and the levonorgestrel intrauterine system (LNG-IUS). A small trial of 41 women demonstrated that the implant was not inferior for treating endometriosis-related pain in comparison to DMPA, but no other studies have been conducted among adolescents. There is limited but consistent evidence that LNG-IUS reduces dysmenorrhea in adults and adolescents. The systemic level of hormone from the LNG-IUS may not be high enough to successfully suppress endometriosis-associated pain. Therefore, it is suggested the LNG-IUS with an oral progestin or estrogen/progestin pill and not the LNG-IUS alone. When counseling on the LNG-IUS, its placement could be done at the time of laparoscopy, to eliminate the possible insertional pain in the outpatient setting [15].

More recently, one compound that seems to have yielded good results without appreciable untoward effects in women aged between 18 and 52 years of age is dienogest [16]. The conventional dose is at present 2 mg daily. Eber et al. [17] evaluated the use of Dienogest in adolescents aged 12–18 years with clinically suspected endometriosis. After 52 weeks of treatment, endometriosis-associated pain improved, along with a decrease in lumbar bone mineral density, which partially recovered after 6 months of treatment discontinuation.

Methyltestosterone and danazol are both exogenous androgens, and they treat endometriosis by inhibiting follicular development and inducing atrophy of endometriotic implants.

Danazol, a 17-a-ethinyltestosterone derivative, has been demonstrated to be just as effective as GnRH agonist in treating endometriosis, but with worse quality-of-life scores reported. Side effects are dose-dependent and typically considered intolerable, such as acne, hirsutism, and weight gain, and maybe permanent, such as deepening of the voice. Transgender male patients with endometriosis may find these side effects desirable, and it can be used danazol for the treatment of endometriosis in transmale clients [1].

If a patient has a suboptimal response to combined hormonal or progestin-only therapies, the provider may consider GnRH agonists such as nafarelin or leuprolide. Continuous GnRH stimulation downregulates the pituitary and creates a hypoestrogenic environment that is highly successful in suppressing endometriosis. GnRH agonists come in many forms, including nasal spray, subcutaneous or intramuscular injection, and implant. The 3-month injectable agonist can improve patient compliance and decrease office visits. The 3-month formulation also provides ample time to trial the therapy beyond the "flare effect," which is when there is initial production of follicle-stimulating hormone (FSH) and luteinizing hormone (LH) prior to downregulation. The "flare" results in a surge of estradiol and causes pain and withdrawal bleeding 21–28 days postinjection. Importantly, it is recommended to limit GnRH agonist therapy to above the age of 16 years because of the potential long-term adverse effects on bone, during a critical period in adolescence for accrual of bone density [13]. For this reason, "add-back therapy" is suggested for all adolescents receiving GnRH agonists, beginning within the first month. Sex steroid add-back therapy aims to decrease the hypoestrogenic effects without stimulating endometriosis. Add-back regimens include norethindrone acetate daily, or conjugated estrogens plus medroxyprogesterone acetate or norethindrone acetate daily. Combination norethindrone acetate (5 mg/day) plus conjugated equine estrogen (0.625 mg/day) add-back seems to be superior to norethindrone acetate alone for increasing bone density and quality of life [18]. Combined oral contraceptives are not appropriate to use as add-back therapy, as they negate the effects of the GnRH agonist. For surveillance, we recommend obtaining dual-energy X-ray absorptiometry at the conclusion of 9–12 months of GnRH agonist use, and repeating bone density testing at least every 2 years if the patient remains on therapy. We recommend discontinuation of GnRH agonist therapy if a decrease in bone density occurs despite add-back therapy.

### 6.1.3 New Pharmacological Options

New medications under active investigation include GnRH antagonists, selective estrogen receptor modulators (SERMs), selective progesterone receptor modulators (SPRMs), progesterone antagonists, aromatase inhibitors, statins, angiogenic inhibitors, and botanicals.

GnRH antagonists may also be considered as an alternative. These agents are a newer class of drugs, available in oral or injection form. They are effective immediately without an LH surge or "flare." The oral antagonist Elagolix is approved for moderate to severe endometriosis-related pain; however, it has not been studied in trials including teenagers [19]. Elagolix is administered as a 150-mg tablet once daily or 200 mg twice a day. Elagolix is not approved as a contraceptive because it does not always suppress ovulation. Furthermore, the incidence of amenorrhea varies widely, from 13.9% to 65.6% in clinical trials; reductions in dysmenorrhea, nonmenstrual pelvic pain, and dyspareunia are observed with this drug [19, 20].

SERMs represent another treatment option through ERa activity suppression, which is essential for endometriosis progression. SPRMs such as asoprisnil, with mixed agonist–antagonist properties suppressing ovulation and endometrial bleeding with antiproliferative effects on the endometrium, have been shown to be effective in inducing amenorrhea and decreasing pain [20]. While aromatase inhibitors block the key enzyme in the extra-ovarian biosynthesis of estrogens, very high dosages to overcome the expression of aromatase are needed, suggesting that they could be more effective as adjuvants to suppress the increase of endogenous gonadotropins with the use of the GnRH agonist. Small studies show pain reduction with recurrence after treatment termination [20]. Botanicals with a possible role in the treatment of endometriosis include the Chinese multiherb Yiweining, which decreases cytokine levels and expression of COX2 and Curcuma, which decreases cytokines and angiogenic factors. Botanicals under investigation include Chinese angelica, red sage root, corydalis, cinnamon, myrrh, peach kernel, frankincense, red peony, persica, prunella vulgaris, and white peony [21].

While current therapies include hormonal agents, new treatments may focus on the inflammatory response in the diseases. The effects on nerves from endometriosis involve physical "entrapment" and chemical "irritation." Both activate immune responses. The immune response to tissue damage and its role in pain has been extensively documented. In endometriosis, not only can there be a response to tissue damage, but the immune response can be altered and indeed dysfunctional, creating a state of hypersensitivity to pro-inflammatory stimuli or molecules [22]. As such, the condition can respond to treatments that target specific immune processes [23]. Consequently, this condition can respond to treatments that target specific immune processes [23]. These treatments involved non-specific immune modulators such as ketamine up to more targeted pharmacotherapies and the current development of novel targets [1]. There is a clear disappointment over the slow progress in the development of new therapeutic agents, and few new drugs have been approved for the treatment of endometriosis in the past decade. At the same time, several experimental drugs have undergone preliminary evaluations and appear to show promising results. One option is to use dopamine receptor agonists (DRAs), compounds capable of activating signaling pathways that lead to changes in gene transcription. In a small clinical study, the administration of quinagolide DRA in patients with hyperprolactinemia led to the reduction of peritoneal endometriotic lesions in two-thirds of cases and the elimination in the other third [24]. Histologically, degeneration was supported by downregulation of the vascular endothelial growth factor (VEGF) and its receptor-2 (VEGFR2), three proangiogenic cytokines, and the plasminogen inhibitor-activator (PAR-1). DRAs reduced inflammation, interfered with angiogenesis, and improved fibrinolysis. Indeed, numerous compounds are capable of exerting anti-angiogenic effects on endometriotic lesions in vitro and in vivo, including progestogens, GnRH agonists, and danazol, although convincing clinical evidence for their efficacy has not been reported [1]. Since the endometrium also undergoes cyclic physiological angiogenesis, it is not clear how angiogenesis can be targeted without causing unwanted collateral damage. Another possible option is the inhibition of histone deacetylase through the administration of valproic acid [25], a pre-prescribed drug approved for the treatment of epilepsy and bipolar disorders. Numerous preclinical studies indicate that this compound is promising and two clinical studies have shown that valproic acid is effective in the treatment of symptomatic and drug-resistant adenomyosis [1]. For both DRAs and valproic acid, large clinical trials have never been conducted. Since these are old drugs and their patents have expired, any large-scale clinical trials are unlikely to be conducted.

### 6.1.4 Surgical Treatment

In a mini-review of dysmenorrhoea in adolescence, Harel [26] state: "If dysmenorrhea does not improve within 6 months of treatment with non-steroidal anti-inflammatory drugs (NSAID) and oral contraceptive pill, a laparoscopy is indicated to look for endometriosis."

In fact, 25–45% of adolescent patients who underwent laparoscopy for chronic pelvic pain had endometriosis and laparoscopy when performed, should not only be for diagnosis but should also include a therapeutic surgical treatment [27].

Pathologic findings in patients with endometriosis visible on laparoscopy are manifold, including the classic endometrial glands and stroma, chronic inflammation, fibroconnective tissue, reactive mesothelial cells, hemosiderin deposition, endosalpingiosis, and adhesions. The natural progression of the disease leads to fibrosis [1].

The endometriosis revised scoring system of the American Society for Reproductive Medicine (rASRM) applied in an adolescent patient can vary widely. In general, no correlation between the stage of disease and the amount of pain experienced was found. Earlier studies tend to demonstrate a higher prevalence of minimal (rASRM stage I) or mild (rASRM stage II) disease. More recently, however, several authors have reported severe (rASRM Stage III or IV) endometriosis in adolescents. Endometrioma has been found in 16–32.7% of adolescents undergoing surgery for endometriosis [28]. In the Dun et al. [2] series, of 25 adolescents with surgically diagnosed endometriosis, most had Stage I (68%) endometriosis, followed by Stages II (20%) and III (12%). None of the adolescents had Stage IV endometriosis. Matalliotakis et al. [29] reported that 22/55 (45.4%) of the adolescents with endometriosis in their cohort had Stage I disease, 20/55 (36.4%) had Stage II disease, 8/55 (14.5%) had Stage III disease, and 2/55 (3.7%) had Stage IV disease. In the Audebert et al. [30] series, 33 (60%) of the cases were classified as Stages I–II, 22 (40%) as Stages III–IV, and 6 (10.9%) were classified as deep infiltrating endometriosis (DIE). Smorgick et al. [28] observed a prevalence of advanced stage (moderate to severe) endometriosis of 23% in women aged ≤22 years at the time of surgery. Overall, the literature on the prevalence of advanced disease varies widely, from 8.1% to 88.9%.

In view of its proven benefits in the adult population, such as less postoperative analgesia and a shorter hospital stay, laparoscopy should be the standard operating technique used in the assessment and treatment of endometriosis in the adolescent patient. Patient positioning during laparoscopy is similar to that used in adults. The adolescent patient must be placed in a dorsal lithotomy position, using the Allen stirrups if the patient is tall enough, with the arms folded to the sides and the thumb oriented superiorly [31]. For shorter patients, a frog leg position can be assumed. In many instances, uterine manipulation can be used, after a cervical dilatation, if necessary. A Foley catheter should be placed to maintain bladder decompression during surgery.

The abdominal entry technique remains at the discretion of the surgeon, although the recommended entry point remains at the midpoint of the umbilicus [31]. It is important to keep in mind that many adolescent patients are smaller and thinner than adults, with a shorter distance between the umbilicus and the underlying great vessels. The pneumoperitoneum should be based on a maximum filling pressure and not on the volume of gas. Adolescents can generally tolerate pressures of 10–15 mmHg [31].

The first surgical treatment is most important, with excision and destruction of all visible endometriosis and lysis of adhesions; all deep infiltrating lesions more than 5 mm have to be excised [32]. Implants can be destroyed via electrocautery, endocoagulation, laser ablation, or excision. Large studies have not been performed in adolescents; however, studies in adults have demonstrated that surgical treatment can provide significant pain relief. In stage I or II endometriosis, there is no difference in pain relief with ablation or excision during laparoscopy [33].

Destruction/ablation for superficial peritoneal disease and excision for deeper lesions that grow through the peritoneum can be performed. There is no data to support the use of radical excisional surgery (also called peritoneal stripping) for superficial endometriosis, and since it may increase extensive adhesive formation, it should not be used in the adolescent population [34]. Rectal "shaving" versus excision and endometrioma aspiration versus cystectomy are associated with an increased recurrence rate [32].

### 6.1.5  Outcome of Surgery

Data on pain improvement or cure rates are limited in adolescent patients with no published comparative trials. However, most adolescents do not require more than one laparoscopy in their lifetime as long as they are compliant with medical menstrual suppressive therapy.

It is not possible to predict in which patient the disease will progress. The main risk factor for recurrence is incomplete destruction or excision, whether it is laparoscopic destruction or excision in stage 1–2 endometriosis [33] or full excision in stage endometriosis 3–4.

Surgery alone is not a definitive and adequate treatment; the recurrence rate is 5% in 1 year, 5–14% in 2 years, and 20–50% in 5 years [35].

In a small study of 20 adolescents, Yeung et al. [36] suggested that, in the hands of a skilled laparoscopist, complete excision of all areas of abnormal peritoneum with typical and atypical endometriosis may be sufficient to eradicate the disease. A statistically significant decrease in dysmenorrhea, constipation, dyschezia, pelvic examination tenderness, intestinal cramping, exercise pain, and bladder pain were reported. The authors investigated long-term outcomes up to 66 months (on the average 23.1 months) of patients who were not specifically advised to take postoperative hormonal suppression. Although the rate of repeat surgery was 47.1%, the rate of recurrent endometriosis at surgery was zero [36].

Rimbach et al. [37] agreed with this surgical strategy but claimed that the possibility of achieving this goal is limited by the difficulty of detecting all foci and the risks associated with radical surgical strategies. A small retrospective series of adolescents undergoing laparoscopic excision of endometriosis showed that 73% of adolescents had no pain or significantly improved after surgery, and 9% had partial improvement with a median follow-up of 65 weeks.

In the study by Dun et al. [2], the mean age at the time of surgery was 17.2 (±2.4) years (range, 10–21), and patients were followed up for 1 year. At 1 year, 64% reported resolved pain, 16% improved pain, 12% continued pain, and 8% recurrent pain. The authors stated that once the disease is diagnosed and treated by a skilled gynecologist, these patients have favorable outcomes with hormonal and non-hormonal follow-up treatment.

A cohort of 20 adolescent patients in New Zealand who underwent laparoscopic excision of endometriosis demonstrated a statistically significant improvement in dysmenorrhea, pelvic pain, and quality of life as assessed by the EuroQol Group's EQ-5D questionnaire after a mean follow-up time of 2.6 years [38].

In the Audebert et al. [30] study of 55 cases, symptom recurrence or persistence after excision or ablation of endometriosis was identified in 74% of adolescent patients with a mean follow-up of 97.5 months. This is similar to the rate reported in the retrospective cohort study by Tandoi et al. [39], which noted a 56% rate of symptom recurrence at 5 years of follow-up of patients 21 years or younger who underwent excision of endometriosis. Moreover, a case series by Yang et al. [40] confirms the recurrence of symptoms after the excision of endometriosis, noting a recurrence rate of 55.6% with an average time to recurrence of 33.4 months, although these patients were also treated with postoperative medical therapy.

In comparison, Shakiba et al. [41] investigated the rate of reoperation as a surrogate marker for endometriosis recurrence after both laparoscopic excision of endometriosis and hysterectomy with or without bilateral salpingo-oophorectomy for endometriosis-associated pain in adults. In the subgroup of patients who had laparoscopic excision of endometriosis, the authors found that the percentage of patients who were surgery-free at 2, 5, and 7 years was 79.4, 53.3, and 44.6%, respectively, which tends to mirror that seen in the adolescent population.

Among patients treated for deep infiltrating endometriosis, a trend was observed for higher rates of recurrence that required repeat laparoscopy. Data on the impact of endometriosis on subsequent fertility in adolescents are overall reassuring with a limited effect on the fertility rate. Indeed 72.2% of adolescent patients desiring pregnancy achieved a successful live birth, with 69.2% of these pregnancies occurring in patients with minimal or mild disease [30]. Fertility rates strongly correlated with the stage of endometriosis and were 75%, 55%, 25%, and 0% for stages I, II, III, and IV, respectively [11].

Despite these results, there is no evidence that surgical intervention for endometriosis in the adolescent prevents disease progression or long-term consequences such as adult infertility.

## 6.1.6   Alternative/Complementary Treatments

There is little evidence of the effectiveness of non-pharmacological approaches to the treatment of endometrial pain [42] and empirically-based, non-pharmacological interventions for the treatment of endometriosis and CPP are rare. It is, however, well known in the literature that CPP is very distressing for women, associated with disability and other mental health conditions, and often involves inconclusive and unsatisfactory medical investigations [3].

Existing psychologically based pain treatment interventions, such as Cognitive-Behavioral Therapy (CBT) or Acceptance and Commitment Therapy (ACT), could be revised to meet the specific needs of women with endometriosis and/or CPP.

CBT has been established as a valid and effective treatment for chronic pain conditions, but CBT studies investigating specific interventions for endometriosis and/or CPP in women are lacking. A range of behavioral and medical treatments addressing CPP in women was conducted and psychological therapies are shown to be effective for CPP; however, in practice, treatment recommendations generally come from single studies, and more research is needed. Nevertheless, CBT interventions have proven to be effective in reducing pain, improving sexual function, managing discomfort, and reducing disability for a wide range of gynecological conditions that are associated with CPP [3].

Endometriosis can adversely affect women and their partners' general psychological well-being, adaptation to relationships, and overall quality of life. Significantly more sexual dysfunctions compared to healthy women were reported in women with endometriosis [3].

Research on psychosexual interventions in the treatment of endometriosis is limited but appears to be effective in reducing endometriosis-related pain and improving associated psychosexual outcomes. In particular, the goal would be to achieve an individualized, couple-centered approach to care, integrating psychosexual and medical management for endometriosis.

Alternative treatments can be helpful for treating chronic pain and merit further research. A recent systematic review identified eight studies on complementary treatments, and the authors concluded that acupuncture has been the only therapy till now to demonstrate improvement in symptomatic endometriosis [43]. A Japanese style acupuncture was identified to be a safe, effective, and well-tolerated adjunct therapy for adolescent endometriosis through a randomized, controlled trial. A multidisciplinary approach to endometriosis, with integrative medicine and non-gynecology providers such as pain specialists, mental health professionals, and physical therapists, is a proposed model of care to improve long-term clinical outcomes and to encourage research.

## 6.2   Conclusions

Endometriosis in adolescents is a challenging clinical problem as it may present with a number of clinical and pathological differences versus adult women. Nevertheless, given the chronicity of the disease, the challenge is to avoid a delay in diagnosis, understand the disease and direct effective therapies at an early age. Given that endometriosis and accompanying CPP is a multi-faceted and complex problem, there is a need for a new approach from a diagnosis and treatment perspective. While endometriosis can be treated by surgical excision of the lesions and/or hormonal treatment, sometimes combined with anti-inflammatory drugs, medical treatments are not curative and approximately 30% of women who undergo surgery report ongoing pain after surgical excision of the lesions. Overall, combined medical–surgical therapy aimed at menstrual cessation results in better long-term symptom improvement, tailored according to the severity of patient symptoms, extent of disease, and compliance.

However, it should be noted that pharmacological treatments, while not curative, can be helpful following surgery and may be an effective strategy to limit the recurrence of the disease. By understanding the neural underpinnings of the disease and risk factors for chronification, research could provide a basis for evaluating novel treatments and potentially lay the foundation for successful personalized, precision medicine to shorten diagnostic delay and maximize successful pain remediation. Further research is also warranted regarding long-term sequelae such as infertility in women diagnosed with endometriosis as adolescents.

In conclusion, the goals are represented by: improvement of diagnosis, careful surgical treatment, increase in medical treatment, follow-up, and improvement of scientific data.

**Conflict of Interest**   None.

**Financial Support**   None.

## References

1. Benagiano G, Guo SW, Puttemans P, Gordts S, Brosens I. Progress in the diagnosis and management of adolescent endometriosis: an opinion. Reprod BioMed Online. 2018;36:102–14.

2. Dun EC, Kho KA, Morozov VV, Kearney S, Zurawin JL, Nezhat CH. Endometriosis in adolescents. JSLS. 2015;19:e2015.00019.
3. Sieberg CB, Lunde CE, Borsook D. Endometriosis and pain in the adolescent striking early to limit suffering: a narrative review. Neurosci Biobehav Rev. 2020;108:866–76.
4. Vercellini P, Buggio L, Frattaruolo MP, Borghi A, Dridi D, Somigliana E. Medical treatment of endometriosis-related pain. Best Pract Res Clin Obstet Gynaecol. 2018;51:68–91.
5. Johnson NP, Hummelshoj L, Adamson GD, et al. World endometriosis society consensus on the classification of endometriosis. Hum Reprod. 2017;32:315–24.
6. Seyhan A, Ata B, Uncu G. The impact of endometriosis and its treatment on ovarian reserve. Semin Reprod Med. 2015;33:422–8.
7. Liu X, Long Q, Guo SW. Surgical history and the risk of endometriosis: a hospital-based case-control study. Reprod Sci. 2016;23:1217–24.
8. Sibiude J, Santulli P, Marcellin L, Borghese B, Dousset B, Chapron C. 2014. Association of history of surgery for endometriosis with severity of deeply infiltrating endometriosis. Obstet. Gynecologie. 2014;124:709–917.
9. Zhang Q, Duan J, Olson M, Fazleabas A, Guo SW. Cellular changes consistent with epithelial-mesenchymaltransition and fibroblast-to-myofibroblast transdifferentiation in the progression of experimental endometriosis in baboons. Reprod Sci. 2016;23:1409–21.
10. Unger CA, Laufer MR. Progression of endometriosis in nonmedically managed adolescents: a case series. J Pediatr Adolesc Gynecol. 2011;24:e21–3.
11. Stuparich MA, Donnellan NM, Sanfilippo JS. Endometriosis in the adolescent patient. Semin Reprod Med. 2017;35:102–9.
12. Steenberg CK, Tanbo TG, Qvigstad E. Endometriosis in adolescence: predictive markers and management. Acta Obstet Gynecol Scand. 2013;92:491–5.
13. Shim JY, Laufer MR. Adolescent endometriosis: an update. J Pediatr Adolesc Gynecol. 2020;33(2):112–9.
14. Kaser DJ, Laufer MR. Norethindrone acetate for hormonal suppression of adolescent endometriosis-associated pain. J Pediatr Adolesc Gynecol. 2011;24:e49.
15. Yoost J, LaJoie AS, Hertweck P, et al. Use of the levonoresgetrel intrauterine system in adolescents with endometriosis. J Pediatr Adolesc Gynecol. 2013;26:120.
16. Schindler AE, Henkel A, Moore C, Oettel M. Effect and safety of high-dose dienogest (20 mg/day) in the treatment of women with endometriosis. Arch Gynecol Obstet. 2010;282:507–14.
17. Ebert AD, Dong L, Merz M, et al. Dienogest 2 mg daily in the treatment of adolescents with clinically suspected endometriosis: the VISanne study to assess safety in ADOlescents. J Pediatr Adolesc Gynecol. 2017;30:560–7.
18. Sadler Gallagher J, Feldman HA, Stokes NA, et al. The effects of gonadotropin-releasing hormone agonist combined with add-back therapy on quality of life for adolescents with endometriosis: a randomized controlled trial. J Pediatr Adolesc Gynecol. 2017;30:215.
19. Taylor HS, Giudice LC, Lessey BA, et al. Treatment of endometriosis-associated pain with Elagolix, an oral GnRH antagonist. N Engl J Med. 2017;377:28.
20. Tosti C, Biscione A, Morgante G, et al. Hormonal therapy for endometriosis: from molecular research to bedside. Eur J Obstet Gynecol Reprod Biol. 2017;209:61–6.
21. Weng Q, Ding Z, Lv X, et al. Chinese medicinal plants for advanced endometriosis after conservative surgery: a prospective, multicenter, controlled trial. Int J Clin Exp Med. 2015;8:11307–11.
22. Pinho-Ribeiro FA, Verri WA Jr, Chiu IM. Nociceptor sensory neuron-immune interactions in pain and inflammation. Trends Immunol. 2017;38:5–19.
23. Symons LK, Miller JE, Kay VR, et al. The immunopathophysiology of endometriosis. Trends Mol Med. 2018;24:748–62.
24. Gómez R, Abad A, Delgado F, Tamarit S, Simón C, Pellicer A. Effects of hyperprolactinemia treatment with the dopamine agonist quinagolide on endometriotic lesions in patients with endometriosis-associated hyper-prolactinemia. Fertil Steril. 2011;95:882–8.

25. Li X, Liu X, Guo SW. Histone deacetylase inhibitors as therapeutics for endometriosis. Expert Rev Obstet Gynecol. 2014;7:451–66.
26. Harel Z. Dysmenorrhea in adolescents and young adults: etiology and management. J Pediatr Adolesc Gynecol. 2006;19:363–71.
27. Mama ST. Advances in the management of endometriosis in the adolescent. Curr Opin Obstet Gynecol. 2018;30:326–30.
28. Smorgick N, As-Sanie S, Marsh CA, Smith YR, Quint EH. Advanced stage endometriosis in adolescents and young women. J Pediatr Adolesc Gynecol. 2014;27:320–3.
29. Matalliotakis M, Goulielmos GN, Matalliotaki C, et al. Endometriosis in adolescents and young girls: report of a series of 85 cases. J Pediatr Adolesc Gynecol. 2017;30:568.
30. Audebert A, Lecointre L, Afors K, Koch A, Wattiez A, Akladios C. Adolescent endometriosis: report of a series of 55 cases with a focus on clinical presentation and long-term issues. J Minim Invasive Gynecol. 2015;22:834–40.
31. Sanfilippo JS, Mansuria SM, Donnellan NM. Surgical problems in the pediatric patient. In: Bieber EJ, Sanfilippo JS, Horowitz IR, Shafi MI, editors. Clinical gynecology. 2nd ed. Cambridge, UK: Cambridge University Press; 2015. p. 576–8.
32. Hogg S, Vyas S. Endometriosis update. Obstet Gynaec Repro Med. 2017;28:61–9.
33. Healey M, Ang C, Cheng C. Surgical treatment of endometriosis: a prospective randomized double-blinded trial comparing excision and ablation. Fertil Steril. 2010;94:2536e40.
34. Laufer MR, Einarsson JI. Surgical management of superficial peritoneal adolescent endometriosis. J Pediatr Adolesc Gynecol. 2019;32:339.
35. Saridogan E. Adolescent endometriosis. Eur J Obstet Gynecol Reprod Biol. 2017;209:46–9.
36. Yeung J, Sinervo K, Winer W, et al. Complete laparoscopic excision of endometriosis in teenagers: is postoperative hormonal suppression necessary? Fertil Steril. 2011;95:1909–12.
37. Rimbach S, Ulrich U, Schweppe KW. Surgical therapy of endometriosis: challenges and controversies. Geburtshilfe Frauenheilkd. 2013;73:918–23.
38. Roman JD. Adolescent endometriosis in the Waikato region of New Zealand–a comparative cohort study with a mean follow-up time of 2.6 years. Aust N Z J Obstet Gynaecol. 2010;50:179–83.
39. Tandoi I, Somigliana E, Riparini J, Ronzoni S, Vigano P, Candiani M. High rate of endometriosis recurrence in young women. J Pediatr Adolesc Gynecol. 2011;24:376–9.
40. Yang Y, Wang Y, Yang J, Wang S, Lang J. Adolescent endometriosis in China: a retrospective analysis of 63 cases. J Pediatr Adolesc Gynecol. 2012;25:295–9.
41. Shakiba K, Bena JF, McGill KM, Minger J, Falcone T. Surgical treatment of endometriosis: a 7-year follow-up on the requirement for further surgery. Obstet Gynecol. 2008;111:1285–92.
42. Wattier JM. Conventional analgesics and non-pharmacological multidisciplinary therapeutic treatment in endometriosis: CNGOF-HAS endometriosis guidelines. Gynecol Obstet Fertil Senol. 2018;46:248–55.
43. Mira TAA, Buen MM, Borges MG, et al. Systematic review and meta-analysis of complementary treatments for women with symptomatic endometriosis. Int J Gynaecol Obstet. 2018;143:2.

# The Etonogestrel Contraceptive Implant as a Therapy for Endometriosis

# 7

Federica Visconti and Costantino Di Carlo

Endometriosis is a chronic estrogen-dependent gynecological disease characterized by the presence of endometrial tissue (stroma and/or glands) outside the uterine cavity, which induces a chronic, inflammatory reaction. Most commonly this involves ovaries and fallopian tubes, and rarely endometrial tissue may spread beyond pelvic organs.

Typically endometriosis occurs in young women, with a mean age of diagnosis of 25–29 years, although it is not uncommon among adolescents, and only 5% of cases are diagnosed in postmenopausal women.

Endometriosis-associated symptoms include dysmenorrhea, chronic pelvic pain, deep dyspareunia, cyclical intestinal complaints, fatigue/weariness, and infertility. In about 25% of women, there are no symptoms. Pelvic pain can range from mild to severe cramping or stabbing pain that occurs on both sides of the pelvis, in the lower back and rectal area, and even down the legs, and in some cases, it may be life-limiting [1].

The exact prevalence of endometriosis is unknown, but estimates range from 2% to 10% of women of reproductive age, to 50% of infertile women, and up to 70% of women with chronic pelvic pain refractory to conventional treatment [2].

Although alternate interesting hypotheses have been suggested, the etiology of endometriosis still remains controversial: immune, hormonal, genetic, and epigenetic factors may be all involved, and several theories have been proposed to explain it. In this regard, an increasing body of evidence suggests that once the endometriotic foci are established, a breakdown in the peritoneal homeostasis occurs: on one hand, peripheral mononuclear cells secrete inflammatory cytokines in early phases as well as angiogenic and fibrogenic cytokines in the late stages of the disease; on the other hand, immune-mediated scavenging systems fail to attack and remove endometriotic

F. Visconti · C. Di Carlo (✉)
Unit of Obstetrics and Gynecology, Department of Medical and Surgical Sciences, University "Magna Græcia" of Catanzaro, Catanzaro, Italy
e-mail: cdicarlo@unicz.it

© International Society of Gynecological Endocrinology 2021
A. R. Genazzani et al. (eds.), *Endometriosis Pathogenesis, Clinical Impact and Management*, ISGE Series, https://doi.org/10.1007/978-3-030-57866-4_7

cells which, consequently, escape from the immune surveillance, implant, and proliferate [1].

The diagnosis of endometriosis, based on the history, the symptoms and signs, is corroborated by physical examination and imaging techniques and is finally proven by histological examination of specimens collected during laparoscopy.

The treatment of endometriosis should be planned according to patients' symptoms, with different options related to pelvic pain and infertility.

Chronic pelvic pain represents one of the main important symptoms of endometriosis. Its management includes both surgical and medical treatments. The surgical approach can remove endometriotic lesions at the moment of the direct pelvic visualization but it cannot affect the pathogenic mechanisms of endometriosis—it is unable to "cure" the disease. This may account for the high incidence of postoperative recurrence of symptoms and lesions [3], supporting the hypothesis that endometriotic lesions may re-form even after radical excision.

The pharmacologic approach aims to suppress ovulation through hormonal treatments. Nevertheless, hormonal treatments for endometriosis-associated pain have several limitations to be taken into account: first of all, these treatments should be administered in a continuous regimen and for a long period (until pregnancy desire). In addition, most of the available therapeutic options presented systemic side effects (e.g., decrease in bone mineral density (BMD), climacteric complaints, and weight gain), which preclude long-term use [4]. However, when side effects or poor tolerability requires the termination of the treatment, pain frequently recurs. As in all chronic inflammatory diseases, prolonged clinical therapy is imperative in endometriosis, and should be aimed at the optimization of clinical treatment, based on suppression and control of endometriotic lesions.

According to the guidelines of the European Society of Human Reproduction and Embryology (ESHRE) [5], hormonal therapies are required in the long-term treatment of the disease. The choice of therapy is based on cost, intensity of pain, age of the patient, desire to conceive, and impact of the disease on work capacity, sexual function, and quality of life.

There are no major differences in terms of efficacy between various hormonal regimens. In particular, a consensus exists on the indication of estro-progestins and progestins as the first-line medical treatment option for the management of endometriosis, with or without surgery, in order to mitigate pain symptoms and prevent recurrences after surgery as a part of a combined medico-surgical management.

Progestins are increasingly and successfully employed as a treatment for endometriosis and their use can be safely recommended to many women with contraindications to estrogens as well as in those who do not tolerate estrogens.

The use of progestins is based on the inhibition of the hypothalamic–pituitary–ovarian axis, leading to anovulation with a relatively hypoestrogenic state, because endometriosis growth and activation are stimulated by estrogen, and both estrogen and progesterone receptors are present in ectopic endometrial tissue. The acyclic hormonal environment, leading atrophy of endometriotic lesions and decreased peritoneal inflammatory markers, also modulating the immune response involved in pathogenesis of endometriosis.

Clinicians are recommended to use progestagens such as medroxyprogesterone acetate, dienogest, cyproterone acetate, norethisterone acetate, or levonorgestrel to reduce endometriosis-associated pain.

Depot medroxyprogesterone acetate (DMPA) is effective in the treatment of pain symptoms caused by endometriosis but in long-term administration may be associated with a decrease in bone mineral density. Studies in adolescents have demonstrated that bone loss is regained after DMPA discontinuation, even in younger users [6].

Cyproterone acetate, a 17-hydroxyprogesterone derivative, has anti-androgenic and anti-gonadotropic properties. Vercellini et al. demonstrated that a low daily oral dose of cyproterone acetate (12.5 mg/day) or a continuous monophasic COC (ethinylestradiol 0.02 mg and desogestrel 0.15 mg) were similarly effective in reducing recurrent pelvic pain after conservative surgery for endometriosis [7].

For many years, long-term therapy with norethisterone acetate (NET-AC), a 19-nortestosterone derivative progestin, has been an effective treatment for pain and discomfort. In 2012, Muneyyirci- Delale et al. [8] in a retrospective study found that NET-AC decreased pain in a highly significant way ($P < 0.00001$) and induced regression in endometrioma size already at 3 months.

More recently, attention focused on dienogest (DNG), a semisynthetic 19-nortestosterone derivative progestin that seems especially indicated in the treatment of women with ovarian endometriomas.

DNG produces a local effect on endometriotic lesions, with little androgenic, estrogenic, glucocorticoid, or mineralocorticoid activity and minimal impact on metabolic parameters [9]. Studies have shown that DNG has both an anovulatory and an antiproliferative effect while inhibiting the secretion of cytokines in the stroma of endometrial cells suggesting a possible direct effect on the cyst wall [10]. Some studies demonstrated a promising ability of this drug in reducing the size of endometriotic lesions and associated pain symptoms, with a favorable tolerability profile, and also a reduction in the size of recurrent endometriomas.

Del Forno et al. [11] compared progestin therapy with DNG or NET-AC in symptomatic patients with ovarian endometriomas, both therapies appears to be effective in reducing the size of endometriomas and related symptoms, with a greater effect on symptoms relief and higher tolerability in women treated with DNG.

An alternative way of delivering progestogens are "long-acting" contraceptives (LARC), such as the levonorgestrel-releasing Intra-Uterine System (LNG-IUS) and the progestin-releasing subdermal implants.

Levonorgestrel (LNG) is a synthetic second-generation progestin chemically derived from 19 nortestosterone; it is six times more potent than progesterone, but also has strong androgenic properties and binding potential to the sex hormone-binding globulin. In addition to the oral formulation, LNG can be administered as an intrauterine system (LNG-IUS).

When administered as an intrauterine device, the main mechanism of action of the LNG-IUS is through its local suppressive effect on the endometrium, including glandular atrophy and decidualization of the stroma. The intrauterine administration of levonorgestrel was studied in patients with rectovaginal endometriosis [12] with a subsequent decrease in dysmenorrhea, pelvic pain, and deep dyspareunia, while the size of the endometriotic lesions was significantly reduced. The local concentration of LNG may contribute to reduce not only patients' discomfort related to endometriosis but also determine increased patient compliance during long-term treatment.

The etonogestrel-releasing subdermal implant has been developed as a long-acting contraceptive device, and it has been recommended to relieve endometriosis-associated pelvic pain [13].

The subdermal implant is a cylindrical rod structure, flexible and biodegradable, that contains 68 mg of etonogestrel (ENG), the active metabolite of desogestrel. After subdermal insertion of the implant, ENG is released slowly and steadily in doses of 60–70 µg/day, which decreases to approximately 40 µg at the start of the second year and approximately 25–30 µg at the end of the third year [14].

The ENG implant prevents pregnancy primarily by suppressing ovulation, but also causes thickening of the cervical mucus so that it becomes impenetrable to sperm, and causes the endometrial lining to become thin and atrophic.

An increasing use of subdermal progestin has been observed in the last years, providing a positive impact in the quality of life (QoL) in terms of general health status and physical status, without effect on libido and sexual function [15].

As a positive side effect, this long-term progestogen delivery system has been shown to improve dysmenorrhea. On the other hand of relevance is the fact that the implant has been shown to be effective in improving symptomatic endometriosis. Among the previously published studies on the effects of ENG subdermal implant in patients affected by endometriosis, Ponpuckdee et al. [16] analyzed 50 women with symptomatic endometriosis. All the patients assessed their pain with the Visual Analog Scale (VAS) before insertion and at 4th and 12th weeks after the insertion. During the study period, improvements in pain severity and menstrual symptoms were observed and 80% of women were satisfied with the treatment.

Ferrero et al. [17] in a retrospective analysis investigate the efficacy of the ENG implant in patients with rectovaginal endometriosis with a positive effect on the intensity of pain.

Yisa et al. [18] described a favorable effect on pelvic pain related to severe pelvic endometriosis in five patients; others reported that its therapeutic efficacy for pain relief is not inferior to that of depot-medroxyprogesterone acetate [19]. Recently a multicenter, prospective, observational study was published, on the effects of ENG implant on quality of life, sexual function, and pelvic pain in women suffering from endometriosis [20]. The authors included 25 women affected by one single ovarian cyst (monolateral) with characteristic of endometrioma at transvaginal ultrasound (TVUS), with a mean diameter $>15$ and $\leq 30$ mm; the presence of dysmenorrhea and dyspareunia.

The ENG implant was inserted between the first and fifth days of the menstrual cycle.

The patients underwent gynecological/pelvic examination before at the study start $(T_0)$ and at 6- $(T_1)$ and 12-month $(T_2)$ follow-up. The investigators interviewed patients on pain symptoms (dysmenorrhea, dyspareunia, dyschezia, and dysuria) using a VAS score $(0–10)$, and they recorded a significant decrease in dysmenorrhea and dyspareunia VAS scores comparing baseline to 6 and 12 months. No significant changes compared to the baseline TVUS scans on the mean diameters of endometriomas were observed.

The impact of ENG implant in the control of endometriosis-associated pelvic pain was evaluated through a noninferiority randomized clinical trial in which women with endometriosis were assigned to use an ENG implant or an LNG-IUS [21]. One hundred three women were enrolled and they were then allocated to use either the ENG implant (n:52) or the 52 mg ENG-IUS (n:51).

Daily scores of pelvic pain and dysmenorrhea were evaluated using a daily visual analog scale. Health-related quality of life (HRQoL) was evaluated using the Endometriosis Health Profile-30 questionnaire at baseline and up to 6 months. The authors' findings indicated that the ENG implant is an effective treatment in women with pelvic pain and dysmenorrhea with an improvement both of the mean visual analog scale that the HRQoL during the first 6 months of treatment, in addition, ENG implant is not inferior to the 52-mg LNG-IUS.

In another study, the authors assessed the serum levels of three biomrkers endometriosis- correlated: cancer antigen (CA)- 125, cluster of differentiation (CD) 23 and endometrial nerve fiber density. They concluded that both contraceptive methods reduced concentrations of serum soluble CD23 and endometrial nerve fiber density ($p < 0.001$); however, CA-125 was significantly reduced only among users of the ENG implant ($p < 0.05$), in the future these two biomarkers could be used to follow up medical treatment of endometriosis-associated pain [22, 23].

The ENG implant seems to be a safe, new, effective treatment for endometriosis, but primary reasons for discontinuation from all studies were menstrual irregularities after implant insertion. The irregular bleeding, involving about two-third of women with ENG-releasing implant, represents the most frequently reported adverse event [12].

Meta-analytic data derived from a systematic review of eleven clinical trials have shown that in women with ENG implant the abnormal menstrual pattern, which causes discontinuation rate includes amenorrhea (22.2%) and bleeding, specifically defined as "infrequent" (33.6%), "frequent" (6.7%), and "prolonged" (17.7%) [24].

However, women should be carefully counseled regarding possible abnormal menstrual patterns associated with progesterone-only drugs [25]. In particular, irregular bleeding seems to be associated with lower body mass index [26].

The ENG implant has the potential for providing long-term treatment of endometriosis but future randomized controlled trials on a large population are needed.

## References

1. Viganò P, Parazzini F, Somigliana E, Vercellini P. Endometriosis: epidemiology and aetiological factors. Best Pract Res Clin Obstet Gynaecol. 2004;18:177–200.
2. The Practice Committee of the American Society for Reproductive Medicine. Endometriosis and infertility. Fertil Steril. 2006;86(Suppl 4):S15660.
3. Koga K, Takamura M, Fujii T, Osuga Y. Prevention of the recurrence of symptom and lesions after conservative surgery for endometriosis. Fertil Steril. 2015;104:793–801.

4. Crosignani PG, Olive D, Bergqvist A, Luciano A. Advances in the management of endometriosis: an update for clinicians. Hum Reprod Update. 2006;12:179–89.
5. Dunselman GAJ, Vermeulen N, Becker C, et al. ESHRE guideline: management of women with endometriosis. Hum Reprod. 2014;29:400–12. https://doi.org/10.1093/humrep/det457.
6. Ferrero S, Abbamonte LH, Giordano M, et al. Deep dyspareunia and sex life after laparoscopic excision of endometriosis. Hum Reprod. 2007;22:1142–8.
7. Vercellini P, De Giorgi O, Mosconi P, et al. Cyproterone acetate versus a continuous monophasic oral contraceptive in the treatment of recurrent pelvic pain after conservative surgery for symptomatic endometriosis. Fertil Steril. 2002;77:52–61.
8. Muneyyirci-Delale O, Anopa J, Charles C, Mathur D, Parris R, Cutler JB, Salame G, Abulafi O. Medical management of recurrent endometrioma with long-term norethindrone acetate. Int J Women's Health. 2012;4:149–54.
9. Kohler G, Faustmann TA, Gerlinger C, Seitz C, Mueck AO. A dose-ranging study to determine the efficacy and safety of 1, 2, and 4 mg of dienogest daily for endometriosis. Int J Gynaecol Obstet. 2010;108(1):21–5.
10. Harada T, Momoeda M, Taketani Y, et al. Dienogest is as effective as intranasal buserelin acetate for the relief of pain symptoms associated with endometriosis–a randomized, doubleblind, multicenter, controlled trial. Fertil Steril. 2009;91(3):675–81.
11. Del Forno S, Mabrouk M, Arena A, Mattioli G, Giaquinto I, Paradisi R, Seracchioli R. Dienogest or norethindrone acetate for the treatment of ovarian endometriomas: can we avoid surgery? Eur J Obstet Gynecol Reprod Biol. 2019;238:120–4.
12. Fedele L, Bianchi S, Zanconato G, et al. Use of a levonorgestrel-releasing intrauterine device in the treatment of rectovaginal endometriosis. Fertil Steril. 2001;75:485–8.
13. Blumenthal PD, Gemzell-Danielsson K, Marintcheva-Petrova M. Tolerability and clinical safety of Implanon®. Eur J Contracept Reprod Health Care. 2008;13:29.
14. Croxatto HB, Mäkäräinen L. The pharmacodynamics and efficacy of Implanon. An overview of the data. Contraception. 1998;58(6 Suppl):91S97S.
15. Di Carlo C, Sansone A, De Rosa N, Gargano V, Tommaselli GA, Nappi C, Bifulco G. Impact of an implantable steroid contraceptive (Etonogestrel-releasing implant) on quality of life and sexual function: a preliminary study. Gynecol Endocrinol. 2014;30(1):53–6.
16. Ponpuckdee J, Taneepanichskul S. The effects of implanon in the symptomatic treatment of endometriosis. J Med Assoc Thail. 2005;88(Suppl 2):S7–10, 56
17. Ferrero S, Scala C, Ciccarelli S, Vellone VG, Barra F. Treatment of rectovaginal endometriosis with the etonogestrel-releasing contraceptive implant. Gynecol Endocrinol. 2019;12:1–5.
18. Yisa SB, Okenwa AA, Husemeyer RP. Treatment of pelvic endometriosis with etonogestrel subdermal implant (Implanon). J Fam Plann Reprod Health Care. 2005;31:67–70.
19. Walch K, Unfried G, Huber J, et al. Implanon® versus medroxyprogesterone acetate: effects on pain scores in patients with symptomatic endometriosis—a pilot study. Contraception. 2009;79:29–34.
20. Sansone A, De Rosa N, Giampaolino P, Guida M, Laganà AS, Di Carlo C. Effects of etonogestrel implant on quality of life, sexual function, and pelvic pain in women suffering from endometriosis: results from a multicenter, prospective, observational study. Arch Gynecol Obstet. 2018;298(4):731–6.
21. Carvalho N, Margatho D, Cursino K, Benetti-Pinto CL, Bahamondes L. Control of endometriosis-associated pain with etonogestrel-releasing contraceptive implant and 52-mg levonorgestrel-releasing intrauterine system: randomized clinical trial. Fertil Steril. 2018;110 (6):1129–36.
22. Margatho D, Mota Carvalho N, Eloy L, Bahamondes L. Assessment of biomarkers in women with endometriosis-associated pain using the ENG contraceptive implant or the 52 mg LNG-IUS: a non-inferiority randomised clinical trial. Eur J Contracept Reprod Health Care. 2018;23(5):344–50.
23. Margatho D, Carvalho NM, Bahamondes L. Endometriosis-associated pain scores and biomarkers in users of the etonogestrel-releasing subdermal implant or the 52-mg

levonorgestrel-releasing intrauterine system for up to 24 months. Eur J Contracept Reprod Health Care. 2020;18:1–8.

24. Mansour D, Korver T, Marintcheva-Petrova M, Fraser IS. The effects of Implanon on menstrual bleeding patterns. Eur J Contracetp Reprod Health Care. 2008;13(Suppl 1):13–28.

25. Guida M, Visconti F, Cibarelli F, Granozio G, Troisi J, Martini E, Nappi R. Counseling and management of patients requesting subcutaneous contraceptive implants: proposal for a decisional algorithm. Gynecol Endocrinol. 2014;30(7):525–31.

26. Di Carlo C, Guida M, De Rosa N, Sansone A, Gargano V, Cagnacci A, Nappi C. Bleeding profile in users of an etonogestrel subdermal implant: effects of anthropometric variables. An observational uncontrolled preliminary study in Italian population. Gynecol Endocrinol. 2015;31(6):491–4.

# Impact of Endometrioma Surgery on Ovarian Reserve

Stefano Angioni, Francesco Scicchitano, Marco Sigilli, Antonio G. Succu, Stefania Saponara, and Maurizio N. D'Alterio

## 8.1 Introduction

Endometriosis is defined as the abnormal growth of endometrial tissue (glands and stroma) outside the uterus, frequently in very distant sites, like the brain or thorax [1, 2]. Clinical presentation of endometriosis varies from chronic pelvic pain to infertility. Regarding the latter, endometriosis is associated with increased production of prostaglandins, metalloproteases, cytokines and chemokines that generate a constant inflammatory process with adverse effects on the normal function of sperm transport, oocytes and embryo implantation [3]. Endometriosis represents more than 50% of female infertility causes and the drop of fertility is related to the severity of the disease [4]. Approximately 44% of patients affected by endometriosis have an ovarian endometrioma (OMA) (Fig. 8.1), which is a cystic ovarian formation, often unilocular (or up to four locations), containing ground glass cystic fluid and with typically scattered vascularity [5]. The appearance of the vascular pattern of OMA, in terms of colour Doppler and Doppler flow indices, seems to be very useful for differentiating it from other lesions of dense vascular distribution, such as corpora lutea or ovarian neoplasms [5].

## 8.2 Ovarian Reserve Markers

The endometrioma effect on fertility is currently assessed through the analysis of two parameters: follicular antral count (AFC) and anti-Mullerian hormone (AMH), which are both positively correlated with the ovarian reserve. AFC is often reduced in women with OMA and some studies have speculated that the cause is the OMA pro-inflammatory effect on ovarian follicles [6]. Other authors have supposed that

S. Angioni (✉) · F. Scicchitano · M. Sigilli · A. G. Succu · S. Saponara · M. N. D'Alterio
Department of Surgical Sciences, University of Cagliari, Cagliari, Italy

© International Society of Gynecological Endocrinology 2021
A. R. Genazzani et al. (eds.), *Endometriosis Pathogenesis, Clinical Impact and Management*, ISGE Series, https://doi.org/10.1007/978-3-030-57866-4_8

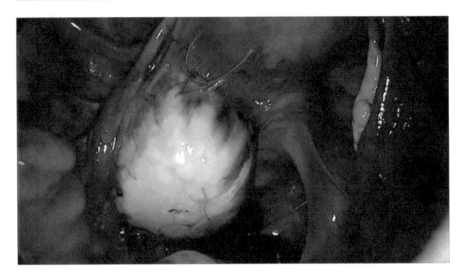

**Fig. 8.1** Left OMA laparoscopic view

OMA may hide antral follicles, which consequently can erroneously appear as reduced on ultrasound examination [7].

AMH is produced in the ovary by granulosa cells of antral follicles. It is released into the follicular fluid and blood vessels, and its levels are measured in peripheral blood. In adult women, its role probably consists of the regulation of folliculogenesis, predominantly in the mechanism of inhibiting primordial follicle recruitment and decreasing the sensitivity of small antral follicles to follicle-stimulating hormone (FSH) activity [8]. AMH has been studied as a possible marker for predicting ovarian reserve and therefore as a fertility indicator, and may also be a very useful predictive marker of the time of menopause [8]. Currently, AMH is the best predictive marker of ovarian reserve since it undergoes fewer fluctuations during the menstrual cycle than other hormones such as FSH, inhibin B or estradiol (E2) [9]. The main clinical applications of AMH determination in women have been the assessment of ovarian reserve in the diagnostics of infertility, premature ovarian failure and hypogonadotropic hypogonadism, as well as in women with OMA or stage IV endometriosis classified by the revised score of the American Society of Reproductive Medicine (rASRM) [10]. Streuli et al. have shown that a decrease in AMH is not significant in patients with OMA and can also be related to other causes, such as age or previous surgery for OMA [11]. As a result, measuring AMH levels could be very useful in predicting ovarian damage caused by surgery [12].

## 8.3    OMA Management

Medical therapy (in particular Dienogest) is considered the first-line therapy in OMA treatment, proving to be a safe, effective and well-tolerated therapeutic option for long-term control of symptoms and reduction of the volume of endometriomas, thus reducing the number of surgical procedures [13]. OMA surgical treatments have an important impact on the healthy residual ovarian tissue, in terms of ovarian reserve, recurrence, chronic pain and quality of life (QoL) [14, 15].

### 8.3.1  Cystectomy (Stripping)

OMA laparoscopic excision using the stripping technique is considered the gold standard among OMA surgical treatments [16]. In a Cochrane review of 2008, Hart et al. demonstrated that ovarian cystectomy allows for pain resolution, a high rate of spontaneous pregnancies and a lower recurrence rate of ovarian cysts when compared to drainage and ablation techniques [16]. The stripping technique requires the identification of a cleavage plane between the cyst and ovarian parenchyma (Fig. 8.2). Muzii et al. analysed the histological composition of OMA, showing the absence of a real cleavage plain with greater difficulty for the dissection of the cystic wall and consequently involving the necessity of extensive coagulation in a very vascularised area [17]. Furthermore, they showed that considering all the sections performed in 70 cyst walls, the mean cyst wall thickness was 1.4 ± 0.6 mm with a layer of endometrium covering the internal surface of the cyst for about 60% of the total (median value with a range of 10–98%), while the remaining 40% is represented exclusively by the fibrotic tissue of the pseudocapsule, with no other identifiable epithelium [17]. Unfortunately, the follicles are tightly attached to the endometrioma's pseudo capsule, risking being removed during the cystectomy or damaged by coagulation, thus reducing the ovarian reserve [18]. This hypothesis was supported by two systematic reviews of Somigliana et al. and Raffi et al., who reported a significant reduction in ovarian reserve, assessed by

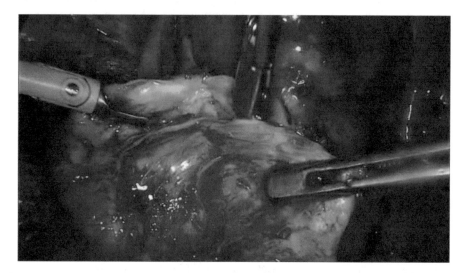

**Fig. 8.2** Laparoscopic stripping technique

AMH-level measurement, after OMA surgical excision [19, 20]. The same results were found by Busacca et al., who showed that patients who underwent in vitro fertilisation techniques after surgery showed greater resistance to hormonal stimulation [21]. The damage mechanism caused by the OMA and its excision can be associated with three main reasons: firstly, the stress related to the presence of the ovarian cyst itself; secondly, laparoscopic cystectomy, also due to the removal of healthy ovarian tissue; finally, haemostasis of the bleeding ovarian parenchyma after stripping, which damages the healthy ovarian tissue and its vascularisation [22]. Haemostasis is a necessary step after stripping and can be done via several methods. Electrocoagulation with bipolar energy is the most common haemostasis technique performed after surgery by many surgeons, although it must be limited to avoid excessive damage to healthy ovarian tissue [23]. Additionally, haemostasis can be performed by suturing, which has the advantage of avoiding thermal damage but, at the same time, requires excellent surgical ability, to obtain the correct tension and avoid the ischemia of the ovarian tissue. Moreover, the materials used for suturing can cause inflammation and post-surgical oedema of the tissue [23]. Litta et al., performing an intracortical suture, found a non-statistically significant reduction in serum AMH levels after surgical excision of the cysts, suggesting that an appropriate surgical technique, without the use of bipolar coagulation of the ovarian edge, did not create a significant reduction in ovarian reserve [14]. In a prospective randomised study, Xiao et al. compared the ovarian reserve in patients undergoing cystectomy followed by haemostasis performed with bipolar energy compared to haemostasis obtained with suture of the ovarian tissue. Six months after surgery, the differences in AFC and AMH between the suture group and the electrocoagulation group were statistically significant [24]. In 2015, Nappi et al. showed another way to achieve the haemostasis after stripping using the dual wavelengths diode laser system (DWLS) [25]. This laser technology involves the use of two wavelengths (980 and 1470 nm), which cause the contemporary absorption of energy in both $H_2O$ and haemoglobin, providing excellent haemostasis, cutting, vaporisation and low thermal penetration [26]. Nappi et al. evaluated AMH levels in the early proliferative phase of the menstrual cycle in three stages: before surgery ($T_0$), after 4–6 weeks ($T_1$) and after 6–9 months ($T_2$) from surgery. The results showed that serum AMH levels decreased significantly in the first month after surgery ($T_1$) and then gradually increased towards the baseline value in the next 6–9 months, remaining at lower levels than the pre-operative AMH value. Their results suggested that an appropriate surgical technique with the use of laser haemostasis did not determine a significant reduction of ovarian reserve, probably because of the possibility of regulating the power and duration of the tissue exposure to the laser [25].

In 2015, Angioni et al. evaluated ovarian reserve after OMA laparoscopic excision, comparing single-port access laparoscopy (SPAL) to multiple-port laparoscopy (MPL); both AMH and AFC were significantly lower in the SPAL group versus the MPL group. Furthermore, surgical times and bleeding are increased using the SPAL technique [27]. The insertion of all the laparoscopic instruments in a single umbilical incision renders the movements more difficult, thereby limiting the possibility of traction and counter traction needed for the excision. SPAL cystectomy should not be recommended to patients who want to preserve their fertility after OMA surgery, even if it could represent a less invasive approach to benign diseases in terms of cosmetic outcome [27].

## 8.3.2 Ablative Techniques

Recently, some concerns have been raised as to the possibility that OMA surgical excision may negatively impact on the ovarian reserve of the operated ovary; in order to avoid excessive removal of healthy ovarian tissue, non-excisional techniques (with cyst wall left in situ and then ablated or vaporised) could represent a less aggressive approach towards ovarian reserve [28].

However, the risk of using a tissue-sparing technique is the increased recurrence rate [29]. Recent studies affirm that new technologies, such as $CO_2$ laser or plasma-energy laser, can better manage the depth of penetration and the amount of heat generated [30].

$CO_2$ laser technology can deliver energy with little thermal spread. This surgical procedure was inspired by the one employed by Jacques Donnez in 1996 in which a $CO_2$ laser was used in the 'three-step procedure' [28]. Tsolakidis et al. carried out a study with the intent to compare OMA stripping to a 'three-steps' ablative technique using $CO_2$ laser [31]. The three steps are: laparoscopic cyst drainage with biopsy and histological examination; medical therapy with a gonadotropin-releasing hormone (GnRH) agonist for 3 months to reduce OMA volume and vascularisation; and further laparoscopy to perform vaporisation of the cystic wall with the $CO_2$ laser. Six months after treatment, an evaluation of AMH levels and AFC was carried out: AMH levels were significantly lower in the in women treated with cystectomy, while AFC was significantly higher in the group treated with the 'three-step' technique [31].

The 'one step' $CO_2$ laser vaporisation procedure consists, during the same surgery, of cystic content drainage, cystic wall biopsy and vaporisation of the internal surface with the $CO_2$ laser [32]. The cystic wall is everted to expose the internal surface of the cyst entirely and is vaporised without the need for sutures. With this technique, the surgeon can selectively destroy the superficial layer lining the internal wall of the cyst without reaching the fibrotic capsule and the adjacent healthy ovarian cortex [32]. The first study that compared cystectomy to the 'one-step' $CO_2$ fibre laser vaporisation (without GnRH agonist therapy) was a randomised trial conducted by Candiani et al. in 2018 [32]. They aimed to evaluate the two techniques in terms of preservation of the ovarian reserve, measuring AMH levels and AFC before the surgery and 1 and 3 months later. The study showed a significant increase in AFC and a stable level of AMH among patients treated with $CO_2$ laser compared to those treated with cystectomy. No recurrence of endometrioma has been reported in both groups, probably due to the short follow-up period [32]. In 2011, Carmona et al. published a randomised controlled trial comparing $CO_2$ laser ablation to laparoscopic cystectomy. They found a statistically significant increase in short-term recurrence rates in patients undergoing laser treatment; however, no statistically significant differences in long-term (5 years) recurrence rate were found between cystectomy and $CO_2$ laser vaporisation [33]. Recently, in 2020 Candiani et al. have published their results on the recurrence rate after 'one step' $CO_2$ fibre laser vaporisation during a 3-years follow-up, showing a recurrence rate comparable to those occurring following cystectomy, with the advantage of being an ovarian tissue-sparing technique [34]. Another ablative technique takes advantage of the PlasmaJet technology, first introduced in 2004. The PlasmaJet device can generate high levels of thermal and kinetic energy through an argon plasma energy source, which can vaporise, coagulate and cut the surface of different tissues. The device behaves similarly to the $CO_2$ laser but does not char the tissue. The results are promising in terms of pregnancy rate and recurrence risk, but there is still no definitive data to justify its use as a first choice over other techniques [35].

### 8.3.3 Combined Techniques

In order to combine the advantages of excisional techniques in terms of lower recurrence rates and the less aggressiveness of the ablative technique in terms of better preservation of the healthy ovarian tissue, a new surgical procedure called 'combined technique' has been proposed by Donnez et al. and, Muzii and Benedetti Panici [36, 37]. The combined procedure is performed first with the stripping technique for the 80–90% of the surface of the cyst, followed by coagulation to treat the last 10–20% of the cyst surface that is attached to the ovarian hilus. Donnez et al. evaluated the combined technique using an ablative method ($CO_2$ laser) following OMA stripping. This procedure proved to not be injurious to the ovarian reserve: volume and AFC of the treated ovary remained similar to those of the untreated counter-lateral ovary [36].

In another multicentre, randomised study, Muzii et al. compared the standard excisional technique versus the combined technique for the treatment of bilateral endometriomas with cyst recurrence rates as the primary outcome and ovarian reserve as the secondary outcome, showing no significant differences between the procedures [38].

In conclusion, further metanalysis and randomised prospective studies are necessary to assess the best technique. However, in the absence of additional evidence from the literature, traditional excisional techniques may still be considered the gold standard approach for OMA surgical treatment.

### References

1. Angioni S. New insights on endometriosis. Minerva Ginecol. 2017;69:438–9. https://doi.org/10.23736/S0026-4784.17.04089-8.
2. Pontis A, Arena I, Angioni S. Umbilical endometriosis primary site without pelvic endometriosis and previous surgery: a case report. G Ital di Ostet e Ginecol. 2014;36:336–8. https://doi.org/10.11138/giog/2014.36.2.336.

3. Gupta S, Goldberg JM, Aziz N, Goldberg E, Krajcir N, Agarwal A. Pathogenic mechanisms in endometriosis-associated infertility. Fertil Steril. 2008;90:247–57. https://doi.org/10.1016/j.fertnstert.2008.02.093.
4. Meuleman C, Vandenabeele B, Fieuws S, Spiessens C, Timmerman D, D'Hooghe T. High prevalence of endometriosis in infertile women with normal ovulation and normospermic partners. Fertil Steril. 2009;92:68–74. https://doi.org/10.1016/j.fertnstert.2008.04.056.
5. Exacoustos C, Manganaro L, Zupi E. Imaging for the evaluation of endometriosis and adenomyosis. Best Pract Res Clin Obstet Gynaecol. 2014;28:655–81. https://doi.org/10.1016/j.bpobgyn.2014.04.010.
6. Halis G, Arici A. Endometriosis and inflammation in infertility. Ann N Y Acad Sci. 2004;1034:300–15. https://doi.org/10.1196/annals.1335.032.
7. Martins WP. Questionable value of absolute mean gray value for clinical practice. Ultrasound Obstet Gynecol. 2013;41:595–7. https://doi.org/10.1002/uog.12449.
8. Broer SL, Broekmans FJM, Laven JSE, Fauser BCJM. Anti-Müllerian hormone: ovarian reserve testing and its potential clinical implications. Hum Reprod Update. 2014;20:688–701. https://doi.org/10.1093/humupd/dmu020.
9. Sowers M, McConnell D, Gast K, Zheng H, Nan B, McCarthy JD, Randolph JF. Anti-Müllerian hormone and inhibin B variability during normal menstrual cycles. Fertil Steril. 2010;94:1482–6. https://doi.org/10.1016/j.fertnstert.2009.07.1674.
10. Yoo JH, Cha SH, Park CW, Kim JY, Yang KM, Song IO, Koong MK, Kang IS, Kim HO. Serum anti-Müllerian hormone is a better predictor of ovarian response than FSH and age in IVF patients with endometriosis. Clin Exp Reprod Med. 2011;38:222–7. https://doi.org/10.5653/cerm.2011.38.4.222.
11. Streuli I, de Ziegler D, Gayet V, Santulli P, Bijaoui G, de Mouzon J, Chapron C. In women with endometriosis anti-Müllerian hormone levels are decreased only in those with previous endometrioma surgery. Hum Reprod. 2012;27:3294–303. https://doi.org/10.1093/humrep/des274.
12. Iwase A, Hirokawa W, Goto M, Takikawa S, Nagatomo Y, Nakahara T, Manabe S, Kikkawa F. Serum anti-Müllerian hormone level is a useful marker for evaluating the impact of laparoscopic cystectomy on ovarian reserve. Fertil Steril. 2010;94:2846–9. https://doi.org/10.1016/j.fertnstert.2010.06.010.
13. Vignali M, Belloni GM, Pietropaolo G, Barbasetti Di Prun A, Barbera V, Angioni S, Pino I. Effect of Dienogest therapy on the size of the endometrioma. Gynecol Endocrinol. 2020;36:723. https://doi.org/10.1080/09513590.2020.1725965.
14. Litta P, D'Agostino G, Conte L, Saccardi C, Cela V, Angioni S, Plebani M. Anti-Müllerian hormone trend after laparoscopic surgery in women with ovarian endometrioma. Gynecol Endocrinol. 2013;29:452–4. https://doi.org/10.3109/09513590.2012.758704.
15. Ceccaroni M, Bounous VE, Clarizia R, Mautone D, Mabrouk M. Recurrent endometriosis: a battle against an unknown enemy. Eur J Contracept Reprod Health Care. 2019;24:464–74. https://doi.org/10.1080/13625187.2019.1662391.
16. Hart RJ, Hickey M, Maouris P, Buckett W. Excisional surgery versus ablative surgery for ovarian endometriomata. Cochrane Database Syst Rev. 2008; https://doi.org/10.1002/14651858.CD004992.pub3.
17. Muzii L, Bianchi A, Bellati F, Cristi E, Pernice M, Zullo MA, Angioli R, Panici PB. Histologic analysis of endometriomas: what the surgeon needs to know. Fertil Steril. 2007;87:362–6. https://doi.org/10.1016/j.fertnstert.2006.06.055.
18. Muzii L, Bianchi A, Crocè C, Manci N, Panici PB. Laparoscopic excision of ovarian cysts: is the stripping technique a tissue-sparing procedure? Fertil Steril. 2002;77:609–14. https://doi.org/10.1016/s0015-0282(01)03203-4.
19. Somigliana E, Berlanda N, Benaglia L, Viganò P, Vercellini P, Fedele L. Surgical excision of endometriomas and ovarian reserve: a systematic review on serum antimüllerian hormone level modifications. Fertil Steril. 2012;98:1531–8. https://doi.org/10.1016/j.fertnstert.2012.08.009.

20. Raffi F, Metwally M, Amer S. The impact of excision of ovarian endometrioma on ovarian reserve: a systematic review and meta-analysis. J Clin Endocrinol Metab. 2012;97:3146–54. https://doi.org/10.1210/jc.2012-1558.
21. Busacca M, Riparini J, Somigliana E, Oggioni G, Izzo S, Vignali M, Candiani M. Postsurgical ovarian failure after laparoscopic excision of bilateral endometriomas. Am J Obstet Gynecol. 2006;195:421–5. https://doi.org/10.1016/j.ajog.2006.03.064.
22. Zhang J, Zhou Y-F, Li B, Jian P, Xiao Y. Influence of various hemostatic methods on ovarian reserve function in women with ovarian endometriotic cyst treated by laparoscopic cystectomy. Zhonghua Fu Chan Ke Za Zhi. 2009;44:583–7.
23. Alammari R, Lightfoot M, Hur HC. Impact of cystectomy on ovarian reserve: review of the literature. J Minim Invasive Gynecol. 2017;24:247–57. https://doi.org/10.1016/j.jmig.2016.12.010.
24. Xiao J, Zhou J, Liang H, Liu F, Xu C, Liang L. Impact of hemostatic methods on ovarian reserve and fertility in laparoscopic ovarian cystectomy. Exp Ther Med. 2019;17:2689. https://doi.org/10.3892/etm.2019.7259.
25. Nappi L, Angioni S, Sorrentino F, Cinnella G, Lombardi M, Greco P. Anti-Mullerian hormone trend evaluation after laparoscopic surgery of monolateral endometrioma using a new dual wavelengths laser system (DWLS) for hemostasis. Gynecol Endocrinol. 2016;32:34–7. https://doi.org/10.3109/09513590.2015.1068754.
26. Angioni S, Mais V, Pontis A, Peiretti M, Nappi L. First case of prophylactic salpingectomy with single port access laparoscopy and a new diode laser in a woman with BRCA mutation. Gynecol Oncol Rep. 2014;9:21–3. https://doi.org/10.1016/j.gynor.2014.05.002.
27. Angioni S, Pontis A, Cela V, Sedda F, Genazzani AD, Nappi L. Surgical technique of endometrioma excision impacts on the ovarian reserve. Single-port access laparoscopy versus multiport access laparoscopy: a case control study. Gynecol Endocrinol. 2015;31:454–7. https://doi.org/10.3109/09513590.2015.1017812.
28. Donnez J, Nisolle M, Gillet N, Smets M, Bassil S, Casanas-Roux F. Large ovarian endometriomas. Hum Reprod. 1996;11:641–5. https://doi.org/10.1093/humrep/11.3.641.
29. Pados G, Tsolakidis D, Assimakopoulos E, Athanatos D, Tarlatzis B. Sonographic changes after laparoscopic cystectomy compared with three-stage management in patients with ovarian endometriomas: a prospective randomized study. Hum Reprod. 2010;25:672–7. https://doi.org/10.1093/humrep/dep448.
30. Roman H, Auber M, Mokdad C, Martin C, Diguet A, Marpeau L, Bourdel N. Ovarian endometrioma ablation using plasma energy versus cystectomy: a step toward better preservation of the ovarian parenchyma in women wishing to conceive. Fertil Steril. 2011;96:1396–400. https://doi.org/10.1016/j.fertnstert.2011.09.045.
31. Tsolakidis D, Pados G, Vavilis D, Athanatos D, Tsalikis T, Giannakou A, Tarlatzis BC. The impact on ovarian reserve after laparoscopic ovarian cystectomy versus three-stage management in patients with endometriomas: a prospective randomized study. Fertil Steril. 2010;94:71–7. https://doi.org/10.1016/j.fertnstert.2009.01.138.
32. Candiani M, Ottolina J, Posadzka E, Ferrari S, Castellano LM, Tandoi I, Pagliardini L, Nocun A, Jach R. Assessment of ovarian reserve after cystectomy versus "one-step" laser vaporization in the treatment of ovarian endometrioma: a small randomized clinical trial. Hum Reprod. 2018;33:2205–11. https://doi.org/10.1093/humrep/dey305.
33. Carmona F, Martínez-Zamora MA, Rabanal A, Martínez-Román S, Balasch J. Ovarian cystectomy versus laser vaporization in the treatment of ovarian endometriomas: a randomized clinical trial with a five-year follow-up. Fertil Steril. 2011;96:251–4. https://doi.org/10.1016/j.fertnstert.2011.04.068.
34. Candiani M, Ottolina J, Schimberni M, Tandoi I, Bartiromo L, Ferrari S. Recurrence rate after "one-step" CO2 Fiber laser vaporization versus cystectomy for ovarian Endometrioma: a 3-year follow-up study. J Minim Invasive Gynecol. 2020;27:901–8. https://doi.org/10.1016/j.jmig.2019.07.027.

35. Mircea O, Puscasiu L, Resch B, Lucas J, Collinet P, von Theobald P, Merviel P, Roman H. Fertility outcomes after ablation using plasma energy versus cystectomy in infertile women with ovarian Endometrioma: a multicentric comparative study. J Minim Invasive Gynecol. 2016;23:1138–45. https://doi.org/10.1016/j.jmig.2016.08.818.
36. Donnez J, Lousse JC, Jadoul P, Donnez O, Squifflet J. Laparoscopic management of endometriomas using a combined technique of excisional (cystectomy) and ablative surgery. Fertil Steril. 2010;94:28–32. https://doi.org/10.1016/j.fertnstert.2009.02.065.
37. Muzii L, Panici PB. Combined technique of excision and ablation for the surgical treatment of ovarian endometriomas: the way forward? Reprod BioMed Online. 2010;20:300–2. https://doi.org/10.1016/j.rbmo.2009.11.014.
38. Muzii L, Achilli C, Bergamini V, Candiani M, Garavaglia E, Lazzeri L, Lecce F, Maiorana A, Maneschi F, Marana R, Perandini A, Porpora MG, Seracchioli R, Spagnolo E, Vignali M, Benedetti Panici P. Comparison between the stripping technique and the combined excisional/ablative technique for the treatment of bilateral ovarian endometriomas: a multicentre RCT. Hum Reprod. 2016;31:339–44. https://doi.org/10.1093/humrep/dev313.

# What Is the Place of Surgery of Deep Endometriosis in Infertile and Pelvic Pain Patients?

**9**

Christian Birbarah, Linda Tebache, Geraldine Brichant, and Michelle Nisolle

## 9.1 Introduction

Endometriosis is a benign chronic gynecologic condition affecting young women in reproductive age and altering considerably their quality of life, causing pelvic pain, dysmenorrhea, dyspareunia, dyschezia, and infertility. It is defined by the presence of ectopic implants of endometrial tissue outside the uterine cavity. These cells are responsible for a local chronic inflammation and in severe stages may distort pelvic anatomy. Several hypotheses have been described to explain endometriosis such as coelomic metaplasia, altered cellular immunity, metastasis, stem cells migration, genetic or environmental factors, or the most accepted theory: retrograde menstruation/transplantation of slouched menstrual blood through the fallopian tubes into the peritoneum [1, 2]. Endometriosis affects 10–15% of women in reproductive age [3]. Pelvic endometriosis can take different forms: ovarian endometriosis (endometriomas), superficial peritoneal implants, and deep infiltrating endometriosis [4].

Deep infiltrating endometriosis (DIE) affects about 20% of women with endometriosis [3]. It is characterized by the infiltration of more than 5 mm of peritoneal tissue with endometriotic lesions [5]. The most common sites of infiltration are the uterosacral ligaments, the recto-vaginal septum as well as the digestive system. Colorectal endometriosis represents the most severe form affecting up to 12% of women with endometriosis and is defined by the infiltration of the muscular layer of the bowel [6]. The main locations are, in order of frequency, the rectum, the rectosigmoid, and the sigmoid [7]. Colorectal DIE is mainly diagnosed using transvaginal sonography (TVS), transrectal sonography, double-contrast barium enema, and Magnetic Resonance Imaging (MRI). The management of DIE is a

C. Birbarah · L. Tebache · G. Brichant · M. Nisolle (✉)
Department of Obstetrics and Gynaecology, University of Liège, Liège, Belgium
e-mail: michelle.nisolle@uliege.be; michelle.nisolle@chrcitadelle.be

© International Society of Gynecological Endocrinology 2021
A. R. Genazzani et al. (eds.), *Endometriosis Pathogenesis, Clinical Impact and Management*, ISGE Series, https://doi.org/10.1007/978-3-030-57866-4_9

real challenge in today's practice. Medical treatment is often insufficient to relieve symptoms and surgery leads to unnecessary complications.

According to the latest European Society of Human Reproduction and Embryology (ESHRE) recommendations, clinicians can consider performing surgical removal of deep endometriosis, as it reduces endometriosis-associated pain and improves the quality of life [3]. However, they recommend also referring women to a center of expertise because surgery in those patients is associated with substantial intraoperative and postoperative complication rates. As for the fertility outcomes, the evidence for performing surgery in moderate to severe endometriosis with the sole intent of increasing live birth is limited. Furthermore, the effectiveness of surgical excision of deep nodular lesions before treatment with assisted reproductive technologies in women with endometriosis-associated infertility is not well established with regard to reproductive outcome [3]. This is mainly due to the lack of Randomized Clinical Trials (RCTs) in the literature. Indeed, one cohort of Bianchi et al. [8] reports higher pregnancy rates after surgery and Assisted Reproductive Technologies (ARTs) but live births did not differ from the ART only group [8]. Another cohort study did not find a beneficial effect of surgery prior to ART [9]. However, these women often have concomitant recurrent pelvic pain and we think these could be good candidates for surgery especially with new data being published suggesting that surgery for deep endometriosis is related to good fertility outcomes. The main focus of this chapter is to evaluate the place of endometriosis surgery in relieving pain symptoms and improving fertility outcomes while reviewing the most commonly used techniques and their complication rate.

## 9.2 Surgical Techniques for Colorectal Endometriosis

Surgery for deep infiltrating endometriosis includes the following: adhesiolysis, ureterolysis, laser treatment, and surgery for bowel endometriosis. The latter can be divided into three major surgical techniques: rectal shaving, discoid excision, and segmental colorectal resection [10]. All three techniques are carried out laparoscopically.

### 9.2.1 Rectal Shaving

Rectal shaving consists of an elective excision of a nodule without opening of the rectal lumen. The dissection is performed by resecting the serosa and the muscularis while respecting the mucosa. It has the advantage of protecting the mesorectum, avoiding the opening of the digestive lumen, and therefore reducing the risk of postoperative fistulas. Shaving is generally carried out using monopolar scissors or ultracision. The main objective is to reach the healthy tissue within the rectovaginal space. In order to achieve this, endometriotic nodules should be dissected from the posterior vagina, the rectum, the posterior cervix, and the uterosacral ligaments [11]. Two techniques can be used.

The standard technique consists of first separating the nodule from the anterior part of the rectum. The deep subperitoneal space located between the uterosacral ligaments and the rectum is longitudinally opened to avoid injury of the hypogastric and splanchnic nerves. Dissection is performed in close contact with the lateral face of the rectum and is directed toward the healthy rectovaginal space located below the endometriosis nodule. Once the lateral walls of the rectum are freed, rectal shaving is performed as deeply as possible into the thickness of the rectal wall in order to remove abnormal fibrous lesions involving rectal layers. The latter can be done by mechanical dissection, the use of cold scissors, or with low thermic energy source ($CO_2$, laser, or plasma) [12]. Thus, the nodule is dissected away from the rectal wall, which then can be progressively mobilized upward. The deep endometriotic nodule is then treated by resection of the vaginal fornix adjacent to the uterine torus (with or without opening the vagina depending on the infiltration depth) and the anterior root of the uterosacral ligaments.

The reverse technique consists first in separating the nodule from the uterine cervix and the affected posterior vaginal fornix [13]. The nodule can then be dissected from the rectal wall.

### 9.2.2   Disc Excision

In the case of infiltration of the entire thickness of the digestive wall, a disc excision could be an option. The nodule can be resected and the intestinal wall sutured in two planes. It is also possible to carry out this resection through transanal staplers. The surgical technique consists of performing a deep shaving which will soften the rectal wall and thus allow discoid excision with the stapling machine. It is of the utmost importance to evaluate the extent of bowel lumen shrinkage before attempting the procedure. If the nodule penetrates deeper than the submucosal layer, the removal of a disc affected by 40–50% of its circumference increases the risk of postoperative stenosis [14]. Two types of anal staplers exist. The first, the transanal circular stapler allows the removal of a nodule measuring up to 3–4 cm and located up to 18–30 cm from the anal margin. The second, the Contour STARR semi-circular transanal stapler, known as the "Rouen technique," is reserved for lesions larger than 3 cm and going up to 5–6 cm, localized at the level of the lower and middle rectum (up to 8–10 cm from the anal margin). It limits resection of the rectum by avoiding segmental resection with low anastomosis and therefore significant amputation of the rectum. The goal is to try to limit the risk of low rectal resection syndrome.

### 9.2.3   Segmental Colorectal Resection

The segmental resection is performed as follows: the right lateral rectal and sigmoid peritoneum is opened from the promontory to the pelvis after locating the ureters. Ureterolysis is performed based on anatomical findings representing one of the major challenges of the surgery. The pararectal fossa as well as the retro-rectal space are secondarily dissected as close to the rectum as possible to preserve the innervation of the lower hypogastric plexus. Separation of the rectum and sigmoid from the posterior wall of the uterus and vagina is then performed. The rectal dissection is continued as low as possible to the pelvic floor. After mobilization of the rectosigmoid and careful dissection of the mesorectum, a section of the rectum under the endometriotic lesion is performed. The distal part of the rectosigmoid is externalized by the mid-suprapubic incision widened to 3–4 cm. After extraction of the rectal stump, resection at an average of 20 mm above the endometriotic nodule is performed. The colorectal anastomosis is then made using end-to-end transanal staplers. The quality of the anastomosis is checked by an intrarectal blue and/or air test [10].

## 9.3    Impact of Surgery on Fertility

"Endometriosis" patients represent a real challenge in ARTs. The mechanism of infertility is yet unknown but is presumably due to multiple factors that include the following: altered anatomy (adherences and tubal disease), local inflammation of the pelvis, altered oocyte quality [15], embryo quality and implantation [16]. Infertility associated with endometriosis is found in 25–50% of patients [17]. Furthermore, the monthly fecundity, normally at 25% per cycle, seems to be reduced by 50% in the presence of pelvic endometriosis [18]. The most common and well-known localization of endometriosis is in the ovaries. Endometriomas' relation to ovarian reserve and thus infertility is well described in the literature. But little is known about DIE and its role in infertility which is the topic of this chapter. The percentage of DIE associated with infertility remains unclear, but we know that DIE represents 20% of endometriosis patients [3]. Its contribution to infertility is therefore not negligible. This is especially true in patients requiring more than two cycles in ARTs as the negative effect of DIE on fertility outcomes has been proved [19]. In the light of this information, new management plans should be considered, alongside with ARTs, to maximize clinical pregnancy rates in these patients. Recent studies have shown that surgical treatment of mild to moderate endometriosis lesions improve both spontaneous and assisted pregnancy rates but do not permit unfortunately to reach fertility rates in non-endometriosis patients.

Does surgery for DIE improve spontaneous pregnancy rates? To focus specifically on the relationship between infertility and DIE alone, all other factors should be excluded. This was effectively done in a retrospective study of Centini in [20] and showed an overall pregnancy rate of 60% in patients given the chance to conceive spontaneously [20]. Couples with endometriomas and sperm count ⩽15 million/mL were excluded. All 115 patients were infertile and had undergone laparoscopic surgery with histologic confirmation of deep endometriosis. The results were very encouraging, as 54.78% of patients conceived, with an overall birth rate of 42.6%. The spontaneous pregnancy rate was 26% and the ART rate 28.7%. More interestingly, there was a significantly higher pregnancy rate in patients undergoing surgical excision of multiple locations of disease. Even if the concomitant presence of adenomyosis could not be separated from DIE, this study showed that the effect of surgery is greatest when performed for the first time in patients with multiple-site disease, irrespective of nodule size and disease location. Although of high value, this study does not take into consideration bowel involvement. In fact, bowel lesions impair normal sexual relation and the idea behind the surgery is to improve spontaneous conception by restoring anatomic function and suppressing symptoms, more specifically dyspareunia. This could allow for more frequent and efficient sexual intercourse. The first study that assessed fertility outcomes after surgery of DIE was the one of Stepniewska in 2010 [21]. The study was conducted on 62 patients undergoing segmental bowel resection for endometriosis lesions by laparoscopy. Those patients had significant stenosis of the intestinal lumen and 50 of them wished to conceive. The total cumulative pregnancy rate was 34%. More importantly, 52% of patients younger than 35 years conceived spontaneously after surgery. Moreover, the difference in recurrence rate between women who conceived (16%) and who did not (12%) was not statistically significant. This has led to the belief that surgical treatment for colorectal endometriosis improves not only pain symptoms but could also help in infertility especially for women with tubal or severe male factor absent. After these results a question arises, are these findings consistent with every surgery route or do they depend on a specific one? One prospective study of Daraï et al. in [22] demonstrated that the surgery route is a determining factor [22]. In his series of 52 patients undergoing colorectal resection, patients were randomly assigned for a laparoscopic procedure or an open surgery. The primary endpoint was the relief of pain, but the study also showed that 39.3% of patients wishing to conceive got pregnant. The overall pregnancy rate at 52 months was 45.1%. Even though not all patients in the study presented infertility, all spontaneous pregnancies occurred in women of the laparoscopy group. The percentage of patients pregnant among those with infertility was 33.3%. The study also emphasized on the timing before pregnancy as two-thirds of the spontaneous pregnancies occurred during the first postoperative year. Finally, these data support that laparoscopic colorectal resection in patients symptomatic and associated with infertility enhances pregnancy even in patients with previous failure of IVF.

Deep infiltrating endometriosis is often multifocal and associated with endometriomas. From this perspective, a prospective cohort study published in 2015 by Roman et al. compared recurrences and fertility among two groups of patients: operated endometriomas with DIE and without DIE [23]. Roman et al. described a high rate of postoperative spontaneous conception after colorectal surgery, suggesting that complex surgical procedures do not impair the fertility outcomes. In fact, surgeons treated all endometriotic lesions including surgery for colorectal involvement (shaving, dis excision, or bowel resection). In the group with colorectal endometriosis, 65.8% got pregnant while only 57.8% conceived in the group without colorectal endometriosis. For the subgroup of patients presumed infertile, spontaneous pregnancy rate was 37.5% while in the total group of colorectal endometriosis a shocking 60% rate of pregnancies were spontaneous. This study shows firmly that concomitant surgery for colorectal involvement in patients with multifocal endometriotic lesions does not have any negative effect on recurrences of disease nor on the probability of pregnancy. On the contrary, it enhances spontaneous pregnancy outcomes. In a study of the same authors published in 2018, they suggested that surgery could be considered as a first-line approach in patients with deep endometriosis infiltrating the rectum and desire for pregnancy [24]. More specifically, it has been shown that women who had been advised to attempt natural conception achieved pregnancy significantly earlier than patients referred for ARTs. Therefore, the surgeon postoperatively recommended either natural conception or ART management based on multiple factors including patients' characteristics (age, parity, antecedents of surgery, ovarian reserve), male sperm characteristics, endometriosis stage, and involvement of ovaries and fallopian tubes. The results were very positive, as 17 patients, out of 36 who intended do get pregnant, conceived naturally (47% of women and 59% of conceptions). In the group of 23 infertile patients, 39% conceived naturally. This study had a total record of 37 pregnancies, among which 65% were spontaneous and 78% delivered healthy babies. The probability of achieving pregnancy postoperatively at 12, 24, 36, and 48 months was 33.4%, 60.6%, 77%, and 86.8%, respectively. All of these numbers could prove that fertility may have been restored by surgery.

One important factor in these studies is worth mentioning: the experience of the surgeon. All surgeries were either done by an experienced gynecologist in deep endometriosis alone or assisted by general surgeons experienced in colorectal surgery. This has led to the possibility of advising patients in matters of fertility based on the findings during surgery. In order to standardize comparisons, create a common language, and facilitate research application, a staging system is then needed for this purpose. The revised AFS (American Fertility Society) system ineffectively predicts the outcome of treatment. Recently, a new clinical tool that offers the possibility to predict pregnancy rates in patients with surgically documented endometriosis who attempt non-IVF conception was validated. This simple scoring system, the Endometriosis Fertility Index (EFI) was done by creating a database with 275 variables, collected prospectively from clinical and surgical data on 579 infertile patients with endometriosis [25]. The data were then analyzed to identify those factors most predictive of pregnancy. The historical factors that predicted pregnancy rates are: age, duration of infertility, and pregnancy history. The least function score, describing the degree of dysfunction on the fallopian tubes, fimbriae, and ovaries was a statistically significant predictor of fertility. It has been shown to be a robust measure of pelvic reproductive potential. Although it was not included in the scoring system, uterine abnormality was also one variable that achieved statistical significance, knowing that only 1 of 9 (11%) patients with a large uterus became pregnant, compared with 4 of 13 (31%) with a small uterus, and 169 of 348 (49%) with a normal-sized uterus. Moreover, deficiencies in the reproductive function of the gametes will affect the prognosis and must be considered separately as fertility factors. Finally, the historical factors, the least functional score, the AFS endometriosis score, and the AFS total score were incriminated in this tool. The EFI is very useful for implementing the right treatment in infertile patients with endometriosis. In fact, it considerably affects the ability to either advise ARTs or spontaneous pregnancy trials.

## 9.4    Impact of Surgery on IVF Results

If surgery has a beneficial effect on spontaneous fertility, why should it have a detrimental effect on IFV results? First of all, the advanced stages of endometriosis decrease substantially IVF pregnancy rates. In addition, data also showed a significant decrease in the number of oocytes retrieved, peak serum estradiol concentration, and fertilization rates in those same patients [26]. To answer questions related to fertility outcomes after IVF in patient managed surgically for DIE, Bianchi et al. divided DIE patients into two groups: Group A undergoing ART procedures and group B undergoing surgery before ART [8]. The choice of enrolment to either group was left for the patient's decision after a full briefing about the procedures and risks. The first results were the confirmation that surgery for endometriomas results in a decreased number of oocytes retrieval and that higher doses of FSH were needed in IVF protocols [8]. However, fertilization rates, the number of top-quality embryos, and the number of embryos transferred did not differ between the groups. In addition, in the group of patients undergoing first-line surgery, significantly higher implantation (32.1% vs. 19%) and pregnancy rates (41% vs. 24%) were observed. This evidence adds to the benefit of surgery that disease removal is associated with improvements in oocyte functional quality and embryo implantation. More importantly, the study suggests the possibility of having underestimated the positive effect of laparoscopic DIE surgery because patients who chose surgery had previously undergone more IVF attempts and had a longer duration of infertility from those who attempted direct ART. In the same concept, an interesting study was published in 2017 by Mounsambote. It consisted of separating people before IVF treatment in two groups: the surgery group and the non-surgery group [27]. Patients enrolled had infertility with DIE without colorectal involvement. The diagnosis of DIE was done by pelvic MRI. The choice of a primary surgery or immediate IVF was guided by the patient's priorities (relief of symptoms or wish for pregnancy). Clinical pregnancy was defined by the presence of a gestational sac with an embryo with positive cardiac activity during a routine ultrasound done around 7 weeks. Patients' characteristics including age, BMI, AMH level, and CFA count were comparable in the two groups. No differences were found concerning IVF characteristics (Total dose of gonadotrophins, number of oocytes retrieved, and fecundity rate). The surgery group had a 40% rate of clinical pregnancy (CP) and the non-surgery group 41%. The total number of CP was 29. There was 11 live birth (31.4%) in the surgery group compared to 12 (32.4%) in the non-surgery group. Patients aged less than 35 years had significantly more pregnancies (79.3% of pregnancies). After three IVF cycles, patients in the surgery group and in the non-surgery group presented cumulative clinical pregnancy rates of 48.6% and 70.1%. Another important aspect of this retrospective study is the low rate of spontaneous abortion (8.3%). Finally, this study demonstrated no negative effect of surgery over IVF results and promoted primary surgery in symptomatic infertile patients, less than 35 years old and without male of tubal infertility. But it does not give answers for a primary surgery treatment in one of the most severe forms of deep endometriosis: colorectal involvement.

In order to suggest the best approach for primary surgery, it is of utmost importance to determine when is best to opt for surgery in infertile women with endometriosis. Who can benefit from surgery and what are the determinant factors? The presence of adenomyosis appears to be a major negative determinant factor of fertility outcomes. Therefore, it seems that fertility results are modest after surgery in patients with concomitant DIE and adenomyosis. Indeed, adenomyosis, age over 35 years and AMH levels below 2 ng/mL were shown to be predictors of low cumulative pregnancy rates in patients with colorectal endometriosis undertaking IVF cycles [28]. Age is an independent factor found in almost all studies done in that matter. We find that it is inappropriate to offer surgery to DIE in patients over 35 years old for the sole purpose of improving fertility. However, in patients with AMH serum levels less than 2 ng/mL, no benefit seemed to be observed after two ICSI-IVF cycles. In this specific setting, surgery with complete removal of DIE should be discussed. Finally, the same study recommends surgery after failure of two ICSI-IVF cycles for patients younger than 35 years with poor ovarian reserve before opting for an oocyte donation program. The main advantage of the study was to demonstrate that pregnancy rates seem to be decreased after the third and fourth IVF cycles in patients with DIE. This seems in concordance with a very recent study of 2019 that shows that in infertile patients with DIE who had had over two failed cycles of IVF/ICSI; complete removal of endometriosis lesions may enhance pregnancy rates by natural conception or ART [19]. In fact, 32 of the 73 women (43.8%) were pregnant following surgery. Almost 22% of pregnancies were spontaneous. The mean timeframe between surgery and the first postoperative pregnancy was 11.1 months. Non-pregnant women had significantly more lesions involving the sigmoid colon and the rectum. Moreover, the non-pregnant group had more history of endometrioma surgery and we already know that repeat endometrioma surgery has a deleterious effect on fertility. Nevertheless, 58.2% of women who already had undergone prior surgery for endometriosis, including cystectomy for endometriomas, but none for DIE or colorectal surgery, were included in the study of Bendifallah that suggested that surgery followed by ART is a good option for women with colorectal endometriosis-associated infertility [29]. This retrospective matched cohort study used a propensity score matching analysis. Each woman who underwent first-line ART was matched to a corresponding woman who underwent first-line surgery followed by ART. To adjust and optimize the matching procedure, covariates were included in the model: serum AMH level, age, and adenomyosis. Results showed primarily that the specific cumulative live birth rate at the first ICSI-IVF cycle in the first-line surgery group compared with first-line ART was, respectively, 32.7% vs. 13%. Secondly, the specific cumulative pregnancy rate at the first ICSI-IVF cycle in the first-line surgery group compared with first-line ART was, respectively, 41.8% vs. 25.5%. Finally, the cumulative live birth rates were significantly higher for women who underwent first-line surgery followed by ART compared with first-line ART in the subset of women with good prognosis factors and women with AMH serum level less than 2 ng/mL. Knowing that the real challenge is to identify the patients who will benefit more from first-line surgery, the study demonstrated that this could be particularly relevant for women with negative factors like low AMH serum levels and adenomyosis.

## 9.5 DIE and Ovarian Reserve: Impact on Fertility Outcomes

IVF protocols and especially FSH doses depend largely on multiple factors. One of these factors is serum AMH levels. While reflecting ovarian reserve, low serum AMH levels were associated with poor ARTs outcomes. Nevertheless, it is of the utmost importance to remember two important things: first, ovarian reserve reflects the quantity of oocytes, and secondly, many studies showed that AMH levels are not predictive of spontaneous fertility.

Keeping this in mind, we cannot but underline the negative effect of DIE on serum AMH levels. More specifically, a retrospective cohort study of Papaleo demonstrated a negative effect of DIE on ovarian reserve [9]. The results were carried out on 51 patients, divided into two groups: ovarian endometrioma group and ovarian and DIE group. While pregnancy rates did not significantly differ in the two groups, the presence of deep disease significantly affected ovarian reserve and the number of oocytes collected. The study however could not determine if the effect is due to DIE alone or to surgery. On the other hand, a newly published data in that matter by Ashrafi et al. in [30] found consistencies that DIE per se is significantly associated with low ovarian reserve and low clinical pregnancy and live birth rate [30]. However, analyzing furthermore the data shows that multivariate logistic analyses revealed that only the Ovarian Sensitivity Index (OSI) and localization of endometriosis were significantly predictive factors for clinical pregnancy and live birth. This means that when OSI (computed as the total number of oocytes retrieved divided by the total dose of FSH administered) drops, the dosage of FSH needed to retrieve oocytes increases, which is a consequence of the bad quality of the oocytes (poor response) and not the reflection of direct quantity of the oocytes as measured by serum AMH levels. This leads us to speculate that even though AMH levels in DIE patients are lower than the general population, it is not necessarily associated with low pregnancy rate and that the latter is impacted by other DIE-related mechanisms as inflammation and bad quality oocytes and embryos.

## 9.6 Impact of Surgery on Pelvic Pain

Pelvic pain is the most frequent symptom in patients with endometriosis. It is the main reason behind the patient's visits to the gynecologist. It is reported that up to 70% of women with endometriosis present dysmenorrhea while deep dyspareunia is reported in approximately 25% [31]. Medical treatment efficacy is only temporary and after 2 months of cessation, the pain reappears. Two RCTs in the literature suggested that pain is improved by surgery. The first compared 32 women undergoing laser ablation for minimal, mild, and moderate endometriosis with 31 women undergoing only diagnostic laparoscopy [32]. Results were significant only after 6 months: 62.5% of patients were better in the laser group. But this study did not include all stages of the disease. The second assessed all stages of the disease and was very similar in design as the previous one [33]. It provided evidence that surgery is successful in treating the symptoms of pain and improving the quality of life for women with endometriosis. However, dyschezia was not alleviated after surgery. This may be due to incomplete removal of lesions especially DIE lesions. Indeed, pain symptoms are related to disease location and proportional to the depth to which the lesions penetrate [34]. One retrospective study that included 132 patients fulfilled all the above requirements and showed that complete surgical excision of DIE lesions is associated with a significant reduction in the intensity of all painful symptoms postoperatively [35]. One of the strengths of this study is its median of follow-up of 3.3 years. What about colorectal endometriosis and pain? The studies are consistent with a decrease in pain symptoms after surgery. For example, the study of Dubernard et al. [36] included 58 women who underwent only segmental colorectal resection for endometriosis [36]. Postoperatively, dysmenorrhea disappeared in 57% of women concerned, dyspareunia disappeared in 51%, dyschezia in 22% and the latter decreased in 56% of women. In addition, pain on bowel movement and intestinal cramping decreased or disappeared in 82.5%. Finally, the most striking result was a significant improvement in quality of life. In the same context, an astonishing review of 49 studies led by Meuleman in [37] confirmed that both pain and quality of life are significantly improved following surgery for colorectal endometriosis [37]. The review also insisted on the need for larger studies with long-term follow-up using validated questionnaires to allow better comparison between the different surgical techniques used and better evaluation of pain outcomes.

## 9.7    Surgery Complications and Their Consequences

One of the reasons for choosing primary ARTs instead of primary surgery in patients with DIE is the fear of surgery complications and their role in delaying pregnancy. Serious complications could have indeed a deleterious effect on the patient's health and could, therefore, shift the surgery primary goals: fertility and pain relief. To analyze the rates of complications, it is important to divide surgery into two distinct approaches: the radical approach that includes mainly segmental bowel resection and the conservative approach that includes shaving and disc excision. In a recent retrospective study on 1135 patients with DIE, deep shaving was the most commonly used technique and represented 48.1% of all procedures [38]. Disc excision was used in 7.3% and colorectal resection in 40.4% of patients. Among immediate complications, recto-vaginal fistula (the most feared complication) was recorded in 2.7% of patients only. More precisely, its rate was 1.3% after shaving, 3.6% after disc excision, and 3.9% after colorectal resection. In addition, the overall rate of leakage of colorectal suture was 0.8% in patients managed with segmental colorectal resection. Pelvic abscess was recorded in 3.4% of patients. Even so, the study could not analyze accurately the relationship between DIE severity and the risk of severe complications, it showed that the rate of overall complications was low and that deep shaving appears to be associated with a statistically significant decrease in rectovaginal fistulae. Also, concerning the shaving procedure, the rate of major postoperative complications was noted to be lower when the reverse technique is used (5%) than when the standard technique is used (22.9%) [13]. In regard to fertility outcomes which is the topic of our chapter, there is still a need for more studies. Nevertheless, one recent study by Ferrier et al. in [39] recorded fertility outcomes in 48 women who had severe complications after colorectal surgery for endometriosis [39]. The median follow-up was 5 years and complications were classified according to Clavien–Dindo classification [40]. Twenty women became pregnant, giving an overall pregnancy rate of 41.2%. More importantly, 80% of the women conceived spontaneously. Regarding the grades of complications, the pregnancy rate was 66.7% after grade IIIa complications and 40% after grade III b complications. The study also found that the occurrences of rectovaginal fistulae, anastomotic leakage, and deep pelvic abscesses were associated with lower clinical pregnancy rates. Finally, the same study emphasized that no woman became pregnant after 6 years and that 65% of the pregnancies occurred during the first 3 years and thus suggested that all efforts should be made to obtain a pregnancy immediately after the initial surgery.

## 9.8 Conclusion

Deep infiltrating endometriosis is still today a debated topic and its management not fully elucidated. Nevertheless, it has been proved that surgery has a beneficial effect on pain relief and improves quality of life. However, this surgery exposes women to the risk of severe complications, such as rectovaginal fistula and therefore should be undertaken in specialized centers with experienced surgeons. Regarding fertility outcomes, while no RCTs have been published in the literature, new emerging data suggests that surgery has beneficial effects on fertility outcomes. In conclusion, the choice of first-line treatment in these women, surgery or ARTs, has to be taken according to the degree of pelvic pain associated with infertility, the age of the patient, the tubal permeability, the ovarian reserve, and the sperm characteristics.

## References

1. Du H, Taylor HS. Contribution of bone marrow-derived stem cells to endometrium and endometriosis. Stem Cells. 2007;25(8):2082–6. https://doi.org/10.1634/stemcells.2006-0828.
2. Giudice LC, Kao LC. Endometriosis. Lancet. 2004;364(9447):1789–99. https://doi.org/10.1016/S0140-6736(04)17403-5.
3. Dunselman GA, Vermeulen N, Becker C, et al. ESHRE guideline: management of women with endometriosis. Hum Reprod. 2014;29(3):400–12. https://doi.org/10.1093/humrep/det457.
4. Nisolle M, Donnez J. Peritoneal endometriosis, ovarian endometriosis, and adenomyotic nodules of the rectovaginal septum are three different entities. Fertil Steril. 1997;68(4):585–96.

5. Koninckx PR, Martin DC. Deep endometriosis: a consequence of infiltration or retraction or possibly adenomyosis externa? Fertil Steril. 1992;58(5):924–8.
6. Darai E, Cohen J, Ballester M. Colorectal endometriosis and fertility. Eur J Obstet Gynecol Reprod Biol. 2017;209:86–94. https://doi.org/10.1016/j.ejogrb.2016.05.024.
7. Chapron C, Chopin N, Borghese B, et al. Deeply infiltrating endometriosis: pathogenetic implications of the anatomical distribution. Hum Reprod. 2006;21(7):1839–45. https://doi.org/10.1093/humrep/del079.
8. Bianchi PH, Pereira RM, Zanatta A, et al. Extensive excision of deep infiltrative endometriosis before in vitro fertilization significantly improves pregnancy rates. J Minim Invasive Gynecol. 2009;16(2):174–80. https://doi.org/10.1016/j.jmig.2008.12.009.
9. Papaleo E, Ottolina J, Vigano P, et al. Deep pelvic endometriosis negatively affects ovarian reserve and the number of oocytes retrieved for in vitro fertilization. Acta Obstet Gynecol Scand. 2011;90(8):878–84. https://doi.org/10.1111/j.1600-0412.2011.01161.x.
10. Nisolle M, Brichant G, Tebache L. Choosing the right technique for deep endometriosis. Best Pract Res Clin Obstet Gynaecol. 2019;59:56–65. https://doi.org/10.1016/j.bpobgyn.2019.01.010.
11. Reich H, McGlynn F, Salvat J. Laparoscopic treatment of cul-de-sac obliteration secondary to retrocervical deep fibrotic endometriosis. J Reprod Med. 1991;36(7):516–22.
12. Roman H. Rectal shaving using Plasma Jet in deep endometriosis of the rectum. Fertil Steril. 2013;100(5):e33. https://doi.org/10.1016/j.fertnstert.2013.07.1973.
13. Kondo W, Bourdel N, Zomer MT, et al. Surgery for deep infiltrating endometriosis: technique and rationale. Front Biosci (Elite Ed). 2013;5:316–32. https://doi.org/10.2741/e618.
14. Abrao MS, Podgaec S, Dias JA Jr, et al. Endometriosis lesions that compromise the rectum deeper than the inner muscularis layer have more than 40% of the circumference of the rectum affected by the disease. J Minim Invasive Gynecol. 2008;15(3):280–5. https://doi.org/10.1016/j.jmig.2008.01.006.
15. Cohen J, Ziyyat A, Naoura I, et al. Effect of induced peritoneal endometriosis on oocyte and embryo quality in a mouse model. J Assist Reprod Genet. 2015;32(2):263–70. https://doi.org/10.1007/s10815-014-0390-1.
16. Minici F, Tiberi F, Tropea A, et al. Endometriosis and human infertility: a new investigation into the role of eutopic endometrium. Hum Reprod. 2008;23(3):530–7. https://doi.org/10.1093/humrep/dem399.
17. Collinet P, Decanter C, Lefebvre C, et al. Endometriosis and infertility. Gynecol Obstet Fertil. 2006;34(5):379–84. https://doi.org/10.1016/j.gyobfe.2006.03.002.
18. Akande VA, Hunt LP, Cahill DJ, et al. Differences in time to natural conception between women with unexplained infertility and infertile women with minor endometriosis. Hum Reprod. 2004;19(1):96–103. https://doi.org/10.1093/humrep/deh045.
19. Breteau P, Chanavaz-Lacheray I, Rubod C, et al. Pregnancy rates after surgical treatment of deep infiltrating endometriosis in infertile patients with at least 2 previous in vitro fertilization or intracytoplasmic sperm injection failures. J Minim Invasive Gynecol. 2019;27(5):1148–57. https://doi.org/10.1016/j.jmig.2019.08.032.
20. Centini G, Afors K, Murtada R, et al. Impact of laparoscopic surgical management of deep endometriosis on pregnancy rate. J Minim Invasive Gynecol. 2016;23(1):113–9. https://doi.org/10.1016/j.jmig.2015.09.015.
21. Stepniewska A, Pomini P, Scioscia M, et al. Fertility and clinical outcome after bowel resection in infertile women with endometriosis. Reprod BioMed Online. 2010;20(5):602–9. https://doi.org/10.1016/j.rbmo.2009.12.029.
22. Darai E, Lesieur B, Dubernard G, et al. Fertility after colorectal resection for endometriosis: results of a prospective study comparing laparoscopy with open surgery. Fertil Steril. 2011;95(6):1903–8. https://doi.org/10.1016/j.fertnstert.2011.02.018.
23. Roman H, Quibel S, Auber M, et al. Recurrences and fertility after endometrioma ablation in women with and without colorectal endometriosis: a prospective cohort study. Hum Reprod. 2015;30(3):558–68. https://doi.org/10.1093/humrep/deu354.

24. Roman H, Chanavaz-Lacheray I, Ballester M, et al. High postoperative fertility rate following surgical management of colorectal endometriosis. Hum Reprod. 2018;33(9):1669–76. https://doi.org/10.1093/humrep/dey146.
25. Adamson GD, Pasta DJ. Endometriosis fertility index: the new, validated endometriosis staging system. Fertil Steril. 2010;94(5):1609–15. https://doi.org/10.1016/j.fertnstert.2009.09.035.
26. Coccia ME, Rizzello F, Cammilli F, et al. Endometriosis and infertility surgery and ART: an integrated approach for successful management. Eur J Obstet Gynecol Reprod Biol. 2008;138 (1):54–9. https://doi.org/10.1016/j.ejogrb.2007.11.010.
27. Mounsambote L, Cohen J, Bendifallah S, et al. Deep infiltrative endometriosis without digestive involvement, what is the impact of surgery on in vitro fertilization outcomes? A retrospective study. Gynecol Obstet Fertil Senol. 2017;45(1):15–21. https://doi.org/10.1016/j.gofs.2016.12. 008.
28. Ballester M, d'Argent EM, Morcel K, et al. Cumulative pregnancy rate after ICSI-IVF in patients with colorectal endometriosis: results of a multicentre study. Hum Reprod. 2012;27 (4):1043–9. https://doi.org/10.1093/humrep/des012.
29. Bendifallah S, Roman H, Mathieu d'Argent E, et al. Colorectal endometriosis-associated infertility: should surgery precede ART? Fertil Steril. 2017;108(3):525–31. e524. https://doi.org/10.1016/j.fertnstert.2017.07.002.
30. Ashrafi M, Arabipoor A, Hemat M, et al. The impact of the localisation of endometriosis lesions on ovarian reserve and assisted reproduction techniques outcomes. J Obstet Gynaecol. 2019;39 (1):91–7. https://doi.org/10.1080/01443615.2018.1465898.
31. Fedele L, Parazzini F, Bianchi S, et al. Stage and localization of pelvic endometriosis and pain. Fertil Steril. 1990;53(1):155–8.
32. Sutton CJ, Ewen SP, Whitelaw N, et al. Prospective, randomized, double-blind, controlled trial of laser laparoscopy in the treatment of pelvic pain associated with minimal, mild, and moderate endometriosis. Fertil Steril. 1994;62(4):696–700. https://doi.org/10.1016/s0015-0282(16) 56990-8.
33. Abbott J, Hawe J, Hunter D, et al. Laparoscopic excision of endometriosis: a randomized, placebo-controlled trial. Fertil Steril. 2004;82(4):878–84. https://doi.org/10.1016/j.fertnstert. 2004.03.046.
34. Fauconnier A, Chapron C, Dubuisson JB, et al. Relation between pain symptoms and the anatomic location of deep infiltrating endometriosis. Fertil Steril. 2002;78(4):719–26.
35. Chopin N, Vieira M, Borghese B, et al. Operative management of deeply infiltrating endometriosis: results on pelvic pain symptoms according to a surgical classification. J Minim Invasive Gynecol. 2005;12(2):106–12. https://doi.org/10.1016/j.jmig.2005.01.015.
36. Dubernard G, Piketty M, Rouzier R, et al. Quality of life after laparoscopic colorectal resection for endometriosis. Hum Reprod. 2006;21(5):1243–7. https://doi.org/10.1093/humrep/dei491.
37. Meuleman C, Tomassetti C, D'Hoore A, et al. Surgical treatment of deeply infiltrating endometriosis with colorectal involvement. Hum Reprod Update. 2011;17(3):311–26. https://doi.org/10.1093/humupd/dmq057.
38. Roman H, Group F. A national snapshot of the surgical management of deep infiltrating endometriosis of the rectum and colon in France in 2015: a multicenter series of 1135 cases. J Gynecol Obstet Hum Reprod. 2017;46(2):159–65. https://doi.org/10.1016/j.jogoh.2016.09. 004.
39. Ferrier C, Roman H, Alzahrani Y, et al. Fertility outcomes in women experiencing severe complications after surgery for colorectal endometriosis. Hum Reprod. 2018;33(3):411–5. https://doi.org/10.1093/humrep/dex375.
40. Dindo D, Demartines N, Clavien PA. Classification of surgical complications: a new proposal with evaluation in a cohort of 6336 patients and results of a survey. Ann Surg. 2004;240(2): 205–13. https://doi.org/10.1097/01.sla.0000133083.54934.ae.

# Endometriosis and Infertility: Surgery and IVF: When, Why, and Outcomes

# 10

Leila Adamyan

## 10.1 Introduction

Endometriosis is defined as a presence of endometrium-like tissue outside the uterus [1]. Every tenth woman of reproductive age suffers from this enigmatic disease. Endometriosis occupies the third place in the structure of gynecological morbidity after pelvic inflammatory disease and uterine fibroids and makes up to 10% in the structure of the general morbidity [2].

Endometriosis is currently recognized as one of the most common diseases associated with infertility. The frequency rate of endometriosis in patients with infertility reaches 50% compared to approximately 6–7% among fertile women with preserved reproductive function.

The problem of restoration of reproductive function in patients with endometriosis-associated infertility is significantly relevant nowadays. Despite extensive knowledge in the field, there is still no consensus on the pathogenesis of infertility associated with endometriosis. The most common etiopathogenetic mechanisms include ovulatory dysfunction and implantation failure, endocrine and immune disturbances, and genetic defects underlying endometriosis [3].

The multifactorial nature of endometriosis-associated infertility can potentially explain the low rate of restoration of fertility in such patients using not only generally accepted (surgical and conservative) treatment methods, but also different methods of assisted reproductive technologies. Development of the most effective management strategy for patients suffering from various forms and stages of endometriosis is one of the top priorities for physicians and scientists.

L. Adamyan (✉)
National Medical Research Center for Obstetrics, Gynecology and Perinatology Named After Academician V.I. Kulakov of the Ministry of Healthcare of the Russian Federation, Moscow, Russia

© International Society of Gynecological Endocrinology 2021
A. R. Genazzani et al. (eds.), *Endometriosis Pathogenesis, Clinical Impact and Management*, ISGE Series, https://doi.org/10.1007/978-3-030-57866-4_10

## 10.2 Endometrial Receptivity in Endometriosis

Endometrial receptivity is a complex of structural and functional characteristics of the endometrium, which determines the probability of embryo–endometrium interaction [4]. Embryo implantation is a multi-stage process involving a large number of cellular and humoral factors. Implantation success depends on two components—endometrium and embryo quality [5, 6].

Previous research has shown that endometrium of women with endometriosis differs from the endometrium of women without the disease. These changes occur at structural and molecular levels and definitely may lead to receptivity disturbance. Changes in endometrium might be an integral part of the pathogenesis of endometriosis-associated infertility.

Most women with endometriosis and concomitant infertility showed impaired gene expression of molecular receptor markers in the middle of the luteal phase. Various researchers have determined impaired expression of more than 100 genes in the endometrium of patients with endometriosis, which affect decidualization and implantation [7].

Increased expression of Wnt7 was among genetic changes revealed in endometriosis. This protein mediates signal interactions between the epithelial and stromal components of the endometrium and causes a violation of cell polarity. Excessive activation of the Wnt/β-catenin signaling pathway during the secretory phase of the menstrual cycle leads to persistent proliferative changes in endometrium and impaired decidualization in infertile women with endometriosis [8].

A significantly reduced expression of NOTCH1 and NOTCH2 was also detected in endometriosis, indicating violations in the NOTCH signaling pathway, which in turn lead to impaired endometrial decidualization [9].

Studies have shown reduced Gal-3 expression in the endometrium of women with endometriosis which impedes embryo–epithelium interaction and delays the proliferation of endometrial stromal cells, which leads to implantation failure [10].

One of the reliable morphological markers of intact endometrial receptivity is pinopodia. These progesterone-dependent membrane protrusions appear in the interval between the 19th and 21st day of the menstrual cycle for a period of no more than 2–3 days. Although their role is still not fully understood, pinopodia appears to be the site of embryo–endometrium interaction, since the blastocyst attaches to the hypothetical receptor on the surface of endometrial pinopodia. The development of pinopodia is associated with an increased expression of molecular receptor markers in the mid-luteal phase of the menstrual cycle. The most reliable markers are leukemia-inhibiting factor (LIF) with its receptor, and integrin $\alpha_V\beta_3$. The possible mechanism of interaction between the embryo and the endometrium is indicated by the presence of LIF-specific receptors on the blastocyst surface: LIF-R and gp130. A direct correlation of the expression of the LIF gene and its receptors with the development of pinopodia has been repeatedly noted [6].

It is believed that $\alpha_V\beta_3$ integrin appears on the luminal surface of epithelial cells of endometrium and embryo during the "implantation window" and continues to be expressed during pregnancy. Many authors suggest a direct correlation between pinopodia growth and the peak secretion of this cytokine [11]. Decreased expression of $\alpha_V\beta_3$ integrin gene was revealed in most women with stage I–II endometriosis and concomitant infertility. It is noteworthy that levels of this integrin returned to normal range in patients with restored reproductive function after treatment with GnRH-agonists or endometriosis excision [12, 13].

It has also been shown that a 5-day therapy with letrozole, a competitive inhibitor of the P450 subunit of the aromatase enzyme, is accompanied by increased expression of integrins, which increases the IVF success rate [14].

Margarit et al. studied the expression of two L-selectin's ligands using monoclonal antibodies and revealed a statistically significant decreased expression in patients with endometriosis [15]. The role of selectins in embryo implantation remains not fully understood. Apparently, they take part in the very early stages of the blastocyst–endometrium interaction.

Many functions of endometrial cells are regulated by cytokine-mediated paracrine or autocrine mechanisms that mediate and modulate the effects of estrogen and progesterone. Interleukin-1 (IL-1), tumor necrosis factor-$\alpha$ (TNF-$\alpha$), transforming growth factor-$\alpha$, endothelial growth factor-1, and colony-stimulating factor-1 are responsible for cell redistribution, regulate the proliferative activity of glandular cells, and transformation of endometrial stromal fibroblasts into decidual tissue.

Inflammation observed in endometriosis setting is inextricably linked to progesterone resistance during the implantation window, increased expression of aromatase and estrogen receptors in the endometrium, as well as the resulting disturbances in decidualization, endometrial proliferation, and implantation [16]. Increased level of pro-inflammatory cytokines, such as $\gamma$-interferon, tumor necrosis factor-alpha (TNF-$\alpha$), interleukins (IL) IL-1, and IL-17 in the endometrium of women with endometriosis have a direct negative effect on endometrium [17].

## 10.3  Tubal Function in Endometriosis

Tubal factor infertility can occur in endometriosis due to alterations in fallopian tubes anatomy. This type of infertility is typically seen with peritoneal endometriosis and is directly related to the severity of the process. Deep infiltrative endometriosis can invade into fallopian tubes' lumen and leads to their obliteration making impossible the passage of germ cells [18]. There is also a functional disturbance of fallopian tubes patency, due to impaired peristalsis of the fallopian tube's wall (decreased contraction frequencies) [19].

Gamete transport is also affected by inflammatory microenvironment which impairs tubal function and decreases tubal motility [20]. Discoordinated contractile activity is observed in endometriosis and linked with exposure to prostaglandins and other biologically active substances that are intensely formed in endometriosis foci, as well as due to absolute or relative hyperestrogenic state and progesterone resistance [21]. Moreover, cyclic hemorrhages in endometriosis foci and the accumulation of serous-hemorrhagic exudate contribute to the deposition of a large amount of fibrin. It can compromise microcirculation, lead to hypoxia, and enhance adhesion formation which can also impair tubal functioning.

## 10.4    Peritoneal Fluid in Endometriosis

Changes in peritoneal fluid composition revealed in endometriosis organize specific environment for ovary, and affect the quality of oocytes. Among different components of peritoneal fluid, researchers actively investigate peritoneal macrophages, since their number, functional activity, and activation potential were found to be significantly increased in women with endometriosis. It is known that macrophages along with endometriotic lesions actively produce various cytokines TNF-α, IL-1, IL-6, IL-8, IL-15, VEGF, IL-10, IL-17, IL-33, IP-10, MCP-1, MIF, RANTES, thus creating the inflammatory microenvironment [22].

Broi et al. suggested that the altered composition of peritoneal fluid during endometriosis causes disturbances in meiosis II, directly affecting the spindle division and increasing the number of aneuploid embryos [23].

Increased incidence of meiosis errors during oocyte maturation was determined during in vitro culturing with peritoneal fluid (1% and 10%) from women with endometriosis compared to women without the disease [24]. In a similar study, no impaired spindle function was revealed during culturing murine oocytes in vitro in media supplemented with follicular fluid of patients with endometriosis. However, an oocyte developmental arrest was detected at the meiosis I division stage, which is caused by activation of the DDR signaling pathway associated with DNA damage. As a result, there is a delay in oocytes' maturation, but not the aneuploidy [25].

## 10.5    Oocytes Quality in Endometriosis

Endometriotic cysts create a toxic environment for ovarian tissue as they contain high levels of proteolytic enzymes, inflammatory cytokines, iron, and reactive oxygen species. Moreover, an increased level of oxidative stress in endometriosis causes oocytes apoptosis while reactive oxygen species compromise ovarian cortex vascularization [26]. Endometriotic cysts also lead to mechanical stretch of ovaries and reduced count of primordial follicles.

Different oocyte dysmorphisms were detected in women with endometriosis including loss of cortical granules, thickening of zona pellucida, decrease in the quantity and quality of mitochondria, and decentralization of chromatin [27].

Juneau et al. studied 1880 blastocysts obtained from 305 women with endometriosis, the control group included 3798 women from whom 23,054 blastocysts were obtained. The results of this study showed that the frequency of detection of aneuploid embryos in women with endometriosis is similar to that in the control group [28].

Despite the fact that the quality of oocytes and embryos is currently evaluated according to morphological criteria, these criteria remain subjective and, as a result, insufficiently accurate. It is necessary to find alternative ways to identify the quality of embryos. The investigation of transcriptional activity in cumulus cells (change in WNT/b-catenin signaling pathway activity leading to atresia of granulosa cells, changes in microRNA expression) may play an important role in the future [29].

Follicles have a metabolically active microenvironment, which includes steroid hormones, growth factors, cytokines, free radicals, and antioxidants along with other elements produced by granulosa cells, endothelial cells, and leukocytes. To a greater extent, a decrease in oocytes quality correlates with an increase in the content of IL-8, IL-12, ADM, while the expression of other pro-inflammatory cytokines is also significantly increased [30].

Myeloperoxidase, one of the markers of oxidative stress found in the perifollicular fluid, can serve as a potential target for attempts to improve oocyte quality in ART programs. When antioxidants were added to the culture media, the quality of in vitro maturing oocytes have improved, which correlated with a decrease in the concentration of myeloperoxidase in follicular fluid [31].

Hsu et al. and Birdsall et al. described mitochondrial dysfunction in granulosa cells of growing follicles in patients with endometriosis, which manifests with diminished ATP production. The authors report that it causes a low metabolic potential of cells and ultimately leads to oxidative stress with subsequent damage to the genetic apparatus of both the oocyte and surrounding cells [32].

## 10.6   Treatment of Endometriosis-Associated Infertility

The question of choosing the most effective treatment method, the feasibility of combining it in the management of patients with recurrent endometriosis, the role and features of ART programs, and ways to increase their effectiveness is still the subject of extensive discussion.

Medical treatment options for patients with endometriosis include oral contraceptives, progestins, aromatase inhibitors, and GnRH agonists. However, hormonal therapy before or after surgery has not been reported to be effective for infertility treatment.

Hormonal therapy prior to surgery is not recommended for women with endometriosis since there is no evidence of a positive effect of hormone therapy on fertility [33].

Hormonal therapy after surgery is also not recommended for women with endometriosis if radical excision of all endometriosis foci was performed [33]. Long-term GnRH agonists use in patients with endometriosis-associated infertility might suppress the expression of implantation factors and lead to decreased endometrial receptivity [34].

There are a lot of different surgical techniques for patients with endometriosis, including laparoscopic or robotic endometriosis excision, endometriotic cyst enucleation, coagulation of endometriotic lesions. There are still a lot of controversies on what should be performed first in patients with endometriosis desiring pregnancy: surgery or any method of ART.

In the case of suspected peritoneal endometriosis, the surgery should be considered only when symptoms are present (pelvic pain, decreased quality of life), and routine laparoscopy should not be performed in patients with unexplained infertility.

Surgical treatment of endometriotic cysts has a risk of ovarian injury via the following mechanisms:

- Removal of healthy ovarian tissue with endometrioma, which might occur due to difficulties in enucleating the cyst or due to inefficient qualification of the surgeon.
- Thermal damage to ovarian tissue by coagulation during endometriotic cyst enucleation which can cause local ischemic changes. Studies have shown that sutures or hemostatic sealants are the better choice than bipolar coagulation in ovarian surgeries [35, 36]. Moreover, ovarian vasculature might be compromised due to aggressive coagulation [37]. All those factors can affect oocytes and cause a decrease in AMH levels and antral follicle count after surgery [38]. Any surgery on the ovaries a priori decreases ovarian reserve, and its degree depends on the type of surgical intervention and increases significantly with repeated surgeries [39].

On the other hand, surgery for endometriotic cysts is beneficial due to histological confirmation of diagnosis and reduced risk of cyst rupture [40].

A meta-analysis of 21 cohort studies demonstrated the negative impact of endometriotic cysts excision on ovarian reserves, including a significant decrease in AMH levels after surgical treatment. In patients undergoing unilateral endometriotic cyst enucleation, serum AMH levels decrease by 30%, compared to 44% in patients with bilateral endometriotic cysts enucleation [41].

Harkiki et al. have reported that laparoscopic resection of mild endometriosis may enhance the ART efficacy [42]. Opposite findings were reported by Tsoumpou who showed that surgical treatment of endometriotic cysts does not affect IVF success rates and ovarian response to stimulation [43].

Surgical treatment is recommended for patients with endometriosis-associated infertility in the presence of a pain syndrome that reduces the quality of life, in case of endometriotic ovarian cysts, and in the absence of the effect of previously performed conservative treatment [44]. Enucleation of endometriotic cyst is recommended to completely remove the pathological tissue, to morphologically verify the diagnosis, and reduce the probability of recurrence [45]. Surgical intervention in patients with endometriosis and infertility may also allow to identify concomitant conditions (inflammation, adhesions, blocked fallopian tubes) and correct them.

Pregnancy planning is possible in 1–2 months after surgical treatment for endometriosis [44]. In the case of blockage of fallopian tubes, the patient should be referred to ART specialist.

Ovarian stimulation can be performed in patients with endometriotic cyst less than 30–40 mm in diameter [46, 47]. Enucleation of such a small cyst prior to ovarian stimulation is not recommended, especially in patients with a history of surgery and verified endometriosis. Several studies have shown that refusing to remove a recurring endometrioma not exceeding 30 mm in diameter before the ART program is time- and cost-effective for patients and avoids the risks of possible complications of surgery, especially with bilateral endometriotic cysts [48, 49]. Meanwhile, other studies prefer to verify the diagnosis of endometrioma with laparoscopy and provide evidence of no decrease in pregnancy achieving rate after endometriotic cyst enucleation [50, 51].

However, surgery remains mandatory in case of suspicious ultrasound findings in women with pelvic pain syndrome. In patients with minimal and mild endometriosis, laparoscopic treatment including excision or ablation of the endometriotic lesions may improve the spontaneous pregnancy rate and live birth rate compared to expectant management [52].

In the study of Vercellini et al., the probability of spontaneous pregnancy within 3 years after surgery in women with endometriosis-associated infertility was 47%, with no significant difference in the pregnancy rate in women with different stages of endometriosis. Within the same timeframe, the pregnancy rate after expectant management was only 33% in patients with moderate endometriosis and 0% in patients with severe endometriosis [53]. In Cochran Database review, laparoscopic ablation of endometriotic cyst was compared to its enucleation, and the last one was associated with increased spontaneous pregnancy rate after surgery [54].

It is very important to follow tissue-sparing techniques in order to protect the follicular reserve of the ovarian cortex during laparoscopic surgical treatment for women with endometriosis. Moreover, all cysts should be enucleated carefully and removed from the peritoneal cavity in Endobag, because the rupture of cyst may cause disseminating of endometriotic cells throughout the peritoneal cavity.

The other important rule is to remove all visible endometriotic lesions, as each remained lesion can increase the recurrence rate of pelvic pain, dysmenorrhea, and dyspareunia.

Both expectant and surgical tactics for endometriotic cysts before ART have potential advantages and risks that must be carefully assessed before making a final decision. Ovarian reserve assessment using AMH and antral follicle count is required before surgical treatment planning in patients with endometriotic cysts [55].

When developing a management strategy for patients with endometriosis-associated infertility, the ovarian reserve, age, duration of infertility, presence of pain syndrome, and the stage of the disease should be taken into account [56].

Patient's age is one of the key factors determining the selection of method of ART. Patients under the age of 35 years may try to conceive naturally (no more than 12 months), or receive GnRH agonists for 3–6 months in addition to surgery, and try to conceive naturally within 6 months after treatment is completed [57]. Endometriosis fertility index (EFI) can also be helpful in developing a management plan for each patient [58]. The beneficial effects of long-term GnRH agonists treatment prior to IVF are mostly seen in patients with severe endometriosis [59].

For women 35 years and older who have not previously received treatment with aGnRH, a long-term protocol of ovarian stimulation is recommended, but the decision is made with regard to the patient's ovarian reserve [60]. The selection of hormonal medications is determined by the patient's ovarian reserve, the endometrial state, and the outcome of previous cycles of ovarian stimulation.

One of the possible options for patients with endometriosis-associated infertility who are preparing for surgery for ovarian endometriosis is to create a bank of their own oocytes/embryos. Such tactics are recommended for patients with diminished ovarian reserve and/or age >35 years. For those patients, the oocyte and embryo cryopreservation can be used as well as ovarian tissue preservation. Embryo cryopreservation is considered the most effective option that leads to a higher IVF success rate. But it could not be used in all patients as it required a large number of oocytes to be present (15–30 depending on the patient's age). Ovarian tissue preservation can be an option of choice for patients who have contraindications for ovarian stimulation [61].

Novel method of "drug-free in vitro activation" is available nowadays for patients with premature ovarian insufficiency (POI) as an alternative to egg donation. Method for activating follicular growth implying surgical intervention was firstly suggested by K. Kawamura, who described in vitro activation of residual follicles by inducing changes in the system of signaling pathways (PI3K-Akt-Foxo3, PTEN). This technology and its modifications are implemented in more than five countries including Japan (Prof. Kawamura), Spain (Prof. Pellissier), and the Russian Federation (Prof. Adamyan) [62]. Studies demonstrate that ovarian fragmentation and reimplantation can lead to changes in gonadotropin and estrogen levels, associated with improved quality of life, obtaining own genetic material in IVF programs. Therefore, it has become possible to restore ovarian function in patients with diminished ovarian reserve [63].

## 10.7 Outcomes of Assisted Reproductive Techniques in Patients with Endometriosis-Associated Infertility

The data on the impact of endometriosis on IVF outcomes is still controversial. According to Senapati et al., endometriosis is associated with lower live birth rates in both autologous and donor oocyte cycles when compared to tubal factor infertility and unexplained infertility [64].

In the study of Somigliana et al., reduced ovarian responsiveness to controlled ovarian hyperstimulation in women with unilateral ovarian endometriotic cysts was shown [65]. Ovarian responsiveness was significantly associated with the size and number of endometriotic cysts. However, retrospective analysis of IVF cycles showed that the number of antral follicles and the total number of oocytes retrieved in women with unilateral endometriotic cysts were not significantly different from those without endometriosis. There was also no association between the size or number of endometriotic cysts and the number of oocytes retrieved [66].

A meta-analysis conducted by Hamdan et al. reported that women with endometriotic cysts undergoing IVF without prior surgical treatment had similar clinical pregnancy rates and live birth rates when compared to women without the disease, but the mean number of oocytes retrieved was lower and the cycle cancellation rate was significantly higher in women with endometriotic cysts [67].

Moderate to severe endometriosis have adverse effects on the outcomes of IVF; however, there is no clear conclusion as to whether to perform surgery on these patients prior to IVF due to the lack of randomized controlled trials, the inconsistent results of previous studies.

According to Hong et al., there is no difference in the IVF outcomes between women with diminished ovarian reserve after endometriotic cysts enucleation and those with diminished ovarian reserve without a history of ovarian surgery [68]. A systematic review comparing ART outcomes between women who had endometriotic cysts with no surgical treatment and those who underwent endometriotic cysts enucleation prior to IVF revealed similar clinical pregnancy rates, live birth rates, and mean numbers of retrieved oocytes [67].

There is no evidence that cystectomy of cysts larger than 30 mm prior to treatment with ART improves pregnancy rates [69]. The effectiveness of surgical excision of deep-infiltrating endometriosis before undergoing ART is also not conclusive, especially in asymptomatic women and symptomatic women whose symptoms are well-controlled with medicines and who are not interesting in pregnancy achievement [70].

According to Vercellini et al., the probability of pregnancy after surgery for recurrent endometriosis seems to be lower than that after primary surgery [71]. In a recent study by Park et al., the numbers of oocytes retrieved after IVF, mature oocytes, and high-grade embryos were significantly lower in patients with two surgeries in anamnesis [72].

## 10.8  New Insights in Endometriosis Research

Currently, there are many studies aimed at identifying biomarkers of endometriosis in blood, endometrium, saliva, and peritoneal fluid. Mass spectrometric analysis revealed significant differences in 15 lipids levels in endometrium and endometriotic lesions of patients with endometriosis which might be potentially useful for real-time endometriosis determination [74]. Studies of endometrial biomarkers also showed very promising results in the differentiation of endometrial samples from women with and without endometriosis. Increased expression of genes FOS, EGR-1, FOSB, DUSP1, ZFP36, JUNB, and JUN was revealed in endometrial samples of patients with endometrioid cysts when compared to endometrial samples of women without endometriosis [75]. Moreover, differentially activated signaling pathways were also revealed in endometrial samples of women with and without endometriosis [76]. Creating a minimally invasive test based on that data will allow practicing physicians to identify endometriosis at early stages and to begin timely treatment. Using novel test-systems will potentially prevent the development of complications of endometriosis, including infertility. Moreover, research is needed to identify any specific and reliable biomarkers to predict the recurrence of endometriosis, which will make it possible to promptly adjust the management strategy and to achieve the most favorable outcome.

## 10.9 Conclusion

Surgical treatment and subsequent intrauterine insemination with ovarian stimulation should be considered in women with minimal to mild endometriosis with infertility.

However, in women with moderate to severe endometriosis, surgical treatment can reduce ovarian reserve and adversely affect subsequent IVF outcomes. According to the recent European Society of Human Reproduction and Embryology guidelines, surgical excision is not routinely recommended before considering ART [73]. Clinicians are advised to assess ovarian reserve prior to deciding whether to surgically remove endometriotic lesions. It is recommended to measure the AMH level at least 3 months post-operatively to create an effective patient-management plan.

Individualized care provided with this in mind to women with endometriotic cysts prior to IVF may help optimize their pregnancy outcomes. Ultimately, the optimal method for the treatment of endometriosis-associated infertility is an individualized decision that should be made on a patient-specific basis. Many factors must be taken into account including but not limited to distorted pelvic anatomy, patient's ovarian reserve, partner semen analysis, age, presence of endometriomas, and length of infertility. Depending on the patient, current treatment options may include expectant management, surgical removal of implants, ovulation induction, or IVF. For women with suspected stage I/II endometriosis, a decision to perform laparoscopy with surgical excision of discovered implants before offering other treatments can be discussed with each patient.

Optimizing and preserving fertility in women with endometriosis begins with preventing iatrogenic injury. Repeat surgeries for endometriosis do not improve fertility outcomes, and patients who do not become pregnant after the first procedure should be counseled to undergo IVF. Patients always should be informed that both the pathogenesis of endometriosis and surgical treatment may affect the ovarian reserve. Moreover, first surgery should become the last one for every patient with endometriosis and it requires effective surgery planning aimed at the most radical endometriosis excision with as less as possible healthy tissue damaging.

## References

1. Koninckx PR, Ussia A, Adamyan L, Wattiez A, Gomel V, Martin DC. Pathogenesis of endometriosis: the genetic/epigenetic theory. Fertil Steril. 2019;111(2):327–40.
2. Wimberger P, Grübling N, Riehn A, Furch M, Klengel J. Endometriosis—a chameleon patients' perception of clinical Symptoms, treatment strategies and their impact on symptoms. Geburdshilfe und Frauenheilkunde. 2014;74(10):940–6. https://doi.org/10.1055/s-0034-1383168.

3. Adamyan LV, Kalinina EA, Kolotovkina AV, Cogan EA. Clinical and embryological aspects of endometriosis-associated infertility. Problem Reprod. 2010;5:47–51.
4. Shurshalina AV. Preparing the endometrium for pregnancy and assisted reproductive technology programs. Consilium Medicum. 2012;14(6):63–6.
5. Niauri DA, Gzgzyan AM, Kvetnoy IM. Immunohistochemical characterics of endometrial receptivity in IVF cycles. Obstet Gynecol. 2014;9:41–7.
6. Adamyan LV, Cogan EA, Kalinina EA, Kolotovkina AV, Fayzullina NM. Morphological and molecular substrate of endometrial receptivity disorder in infertile patients with external genital endometriosis. Obstet Gynecol. 2014;8:45–52.
7. Lessey BA, Kim JJ. Endometrial receptivity in the eutopic endometrium of women with endometriosis: it is affected, and let me show you why. Fertil Steril. 2017;108(1):19–27. https://doi.org/10.1016/j.fertnstert.2017.05.031.
8. Matsuzaki S, Darcha C. Involvement of the Wnt/β-catenin signaling pathway in the cellular and molecular mechanisms of fibrosis in endometriosis. PLoS One. 2013;8(10):e76808. https://doi.org/10.1371/journal.pone.0076808.
9. Su R-W, Strug MR, Joshi NR, Jeong J-W, Miele L, Lessey BA, Young SL, Fazleabas AT. Decreased notch pathway signaling in the endometrium of women with endometriosis impairs decidualization. J Clin Endocrinol Metab. 2015;100(10):E433–42. https://doi.org/10.1210/jc.2014-3720.
10. Yang H, Yin J, Ficarrotta K, Hsu SH, Zhang W, Cheng C. Aberrant expression and hormonal regulation of Galectin-3 in endometriosis women with infertility. J Endocrinol Investig. 2016;39(7):785–91. https://doi.org/10.1007/s40618-016-0435-7.
11. Garrido-Gómez T, Ruiz-Alonso M, Blesa D, Diaz-Gimeno P, Vilella F, Simón C. Profiling the gene signature of endometrial re- ceptivity: clinical results. Fertil Steril. 2013;4:1078–85. https://doi.org/10.1016/j.fertnstert.2012.12.005.
12. Gauché-Cazalis C, Koskas M, Cohen Scali S, Luton D, Yazbeck C. Endometriosis and implantation: myths and facts. Middle East Fert Soc J. 2012;17(2):79–81. https://doi.org/10.1016/j.mefs.2012.04.002.
13. Xiao Y, Li T, Xia E, Yang X, Sun X, Zhou Y. Expression of integrin β3 and osteopontin in the eutopic endometrium of adenomyosis during the implantation window. Eur J Obstet Gynecol Reprod Biol. 2013;170(2):419–22. https://doi.org/10.1016/j.ejogrb.2013.05.007.
14. Miller PB, Parnell B, Bushnell G, Tallman N, Forstein D, Higdon HL, Kitawaki J, Lessey B. Endometrial receptivity defects during IVF cycles with and without letrozole. Hum Reprod. 2012;27(3):881–8. https://doi.org/10.1093/humrep/der452.
15. Margarit L, Gonzalez D, Lewis PD, Hopkins L, Davies C, Conlan RS, Joels L, White JO. L-selectin ligands in human endometrium: comparison of fertile and infertile subjects. Hum Reprod. 2009;24(11):2767–77. https://doi.org/10.1093/humrep/der247.
16. Fox C, Morin S, Jeong J-W, Scott RT Jr, Lessey BA. Local and systemic factors and implantation: what is the evidence? Fertil Steril. 2016;105(4):873–84. https://doi.org/10.1016/j.fertnstert.2016.02.018.
17. Heublein S, Vrekoussis T, Kuhn C, Friese K, Makrigiannakis A, Mayr D, Lenhard M, Jeschke U. Inducers of G-protein coupled estrogen receptor (GPER) in endometriosis: potential implications for macro- phages and follicle maturation. J Reprod Immunol. 2013;97:95–103. https://doi.org/10.1016/j.jri.2012.10.013.
18. Orazov MR, Radzinsky VE, Khamoshina MB, et al. Effectiveness of treatment of infertility associated with recurrent external genital endometriosis. Gynecology. 2019;21(1):38–43. https://doi.org/10.26442/20795696.2019.1.190230.
19. Xia W, Zhang D, Ouyang J, et al. Effects of pelvic endometriosis and adenomyosis on ciliary beat frequency and muscular contractions in the human fallopian tube. Reprod Biol Endocrinol. 2018;16(1):48. https://doi.org/10.1186/s12958-018-0361-y.
20. Holoch KJ, Lessey BA. Endometriosis and infertility. Clin Obstet Gynecol. 2010;53(2):429–38.
21. Krasnopol'skaia KV. Lechenie besplodiia pri endometrioze. Moscow: Vzgliad Reproduktologa; 2019. p. 28–80; (in Russian)

22. Ahn SH, Edwards AK, Singh SS, Young SL, Lessey BA, Tayade C. IL-17A contributes to the pathogenesis of endometriosis by trig- Gering proinflammatory cytokines and angiogenic growth factors. J Immunol. 2015;195(6):2591–600. https://doi.org/10.4049/jimmunol. 1501138.

23. Da Broi MG, Malvezzi H, Paz CC, Ferriani RA, Navarro PA. Follicular fluid from infertile women with mild endometriosis may compromise the meiotic spindles of bovine metaphase II oocytes. Hum Reprod. 2014;29:315–23. https://doi.org/10.1093/humrep/det37.

24. Jianini BTGM, Giorgi VSI, Da Broi MG, de Paz CCP, Rosa E, Silva JC, Ferriani RA, Navarro PA. Peritoneal fluid from infertile women with minimal/mild endometriosis compromises the meiotic spindle of metaphase ii bovine oocytes: a pilot study. Reprod Sci. 2017;24(9):1304–11. https://doi.org/10.1177/1933719116687658.

25. Hamdan M, Jones KT, Cheong Y, Lane SI. The sensitivity of the DNA damage checkpoint prevents oocyte maturation in endometriosis. Sci Rep. 2016;6:36994. https://doi.org/10.1038/srep36994.

26. Park HJ, Kim H, Lee GH, Yoon TK, Lee WS. Could surgical management improve the IVF outcomes in infertile women with endometrioma?: a review. Obstet Gynecol Sci. 2019;62(1):1–10. https://doi.org/10.5468/ogs.2019.62.1.1.

27. Ceviren AK, Ozcelik NT, Urfan A, Donmez L, Isikoglu M. Characteristic cytoplasmic morphology of oocytes in endometriosis patients and its effect on the outcome of assisted reproduction treatments cycles. IVF Lite. 2014;1:88–93. https://doi.org/10.4103/2348-2907.140123.

28. Juneau C, Kraus E, Werner M, Franasiak J, Morin S, Patounakis G, Molinaro T, de Ziegler D, Scott RT, American Society for Reproductive Medicine. Patients with endometriosis have aneuploidy rates equivalent to their age-matched peers in the in vitro fertilization population. Fertil Steril. 2017;108(2):284–8. https://doi.org/10.1016/j.fertnstert.2017.05.038.

29. Russell DL, Gilchrist RB, Brown HM, Thompson JG. Bidirec- tional communication between cumulus cells and the oocyte: old hands and new players? Theriogenology. 2016;86(1):62–8. https://doi.org/10.1016/j.theriogenology.2016.04.019.

30. Singh AK, Dutta M, Chattopadhyay R, Chakravarty B, Chaudhury K. Intrafollicular interleukin-8, interleukin-12, and adrenomedullin are the promising prognostic markers of oocyte and embryo quality in women with endometriosis. J Assist Reprod Genet. 2016;33(10):1363–72. https://doi.org/10.1007/s10815-016-0782-5.

31. Santanam N, Zoneraich N, Parthasarathy S. Myeloperoxidase as a potential target in women with endometriosis undergoing IVF. Reprod Sci. 2017;24(4):619–26. https://doi.org/10.1177/1933719116667225.

32. Hsu AL, Townsend PM, Oehninger S, Castora FJ. Endometriosis may be associated with mitochondrial dysfunction in cumulus cells from subjects undergoing in vitro fertilization-intracytoplasmic sperm injection, as reflected by decreased adenosine triphosphate production. Fertil Steril. 2015;103(2):347–52. https://doi.org/10.1016/j.fertnstert.2014.11.002.

33. Sroga JM, Montville CP, Aubuchon M, Williams DB, Thomas MA. Effect of delayed versus immediate embryo transfer catheter removal on pregnancy outcomes during fresh cycles. Fertil Steril. 2010;93(6):2088–90.

34. Ruan HC, Zhu XM, Luo Q, Liu AX, Qian YL, Zhou CY, et al. Ovarian stimulation with GnRH agonist, but not GnRH antagonist, partially restores the expression of endometrial integrin β3 and leukaemia-inhibitory factor and improves uterine receptivity in mice. Hum Reprod. 2006;21:2521–9.

35. Ata B, Turkgeldi E, Seyhan A, Urman B. Effect of hemostatic method on ovarian reserve following laparoscopic endometrioma excision: comparison of suture, hemostatic sealant, and bipolar dessication: a systematic review and meta-analysis. J Minim Invasive Gynecol. 2015;22:363–72.

36. Seyhan A, Ata B, Uncu G. The impact of endometriosis and its treatment on ovarian reserve. Semin Reprod Med. 2015;33:422–8.

37. Goodman LR, Goldberg JM, Flyckt RL, Gupta M, Harwalker J, Falcone T. Effect of surgery on ovarian reserve in women with endometriomas, endometriosis and controls. Am J Obstet Gynecol. 2016;215:589.
38. Chang HJ, Han SH, Lee JR, Jee BC, Lee BI, Suh CS, et al. Impact of laparoscopic cystectomy on ovarian reserve: serial changes of serum anti-Mullerian hormone levels. Fertil Steril. 2010;94:343–9.
39. Muzii L, Di Tucci C, Di Feliciantonio M, Marchetti C, Perniola G, Panici PB. The effect of surgery for endometrioma on ovarian reserve evaluated by antral follicle count: a systematic review and meta-analysis. Hum Reprod. 2014;29(10):2190–8.
40. Lee D, Kim SK, Lee JR, Jee BC. Management of endometriosis-related infertility: considerations and treatment options. Clin Exp Reprod Med. 2020;47(1):1–11. https://doi.org/10.5653/cerm.2019.02971.
41. Raffi F, Metwally M, Amer S. The impact of excision of ovarian endometrioma on ovarian reserve: a systematic review and meta-analysis. J Clin Endocrinol Metab. 2012;97(9):3146–54.
42. Härkki P, Tiitinen A, Ylikorkala O. Endometriosis and assisted reproduction techniques. Ann N Y Acad Sci. 2010;1205:207–13.
43. Tsoumpou I, Kyrgiou M, Gelbaya TA, Nardo LG. The effect of surgical treatment for endometrioma on in vitro fertilization outcomes: a systematic review and meta- analysis. Fertil Steril. 2009;92:75–87.
44. Xiao Z, Zhou X, Xu W, Yang J, Xie Q. Natural cycle is superior to hormone replacement therapy cycle for vitrificated-preserved frozen-thawed embryo transfer. Syst Biol Reprod Med. 2012;58(2):107–12.
45. Verheyen G, Tournaye H, Staessen C, De Vos A, Vandervorst M, Van Steirteghem A. Controlled comparison of conventional in-vitro fertilization and intracytoplasmic sperm injection in patients with asthenozoospermia. Hum Reprod. 1999;14(9):2313–9.
46. Brown J, Buckingham K, Buckett W, Abou-Setta AM. Ultrasound versus "clinical touch" for catheter guidance during embryo transfer in women. Cochrane Database Syst Rev. 2016;3: CD006107.
47. ESHRE Capri Workshop Group. Intracytoplasmic sperm injection (ICSI) in 2006: evidence and evolution. Hum Reprod Update. 2007;13(6):515–26.
48. Geber S, Ferreira DP, Spyer Prates LFV, Sales L, Sampaio M. Effects of previous ovarian surgery for endometriosis on the outcome of assisted reproduction treatment. Reprod Biomed Online [Internet]. 2002;5(2):162–6.
49. Somigliana E, Arnoldi M, Benaglia L, Iemmello R, Nicolosi AE, Ragni G. IVF-ICSI outcome in women operated on for bilateral endometriomas. Hum Reprod [Internet]. 2008;23 (7):1526–30.
50. Yu H-T, Huang H-Y, Tseng H-J, Wang C-J, Lee C-L, Soong Y-K. Bilaterality of ovarian endometriomas does not affect the outcome of in vitro fertilization/intracytoplasmic sperm injection in infertile women after laparoscopic cystectomy. Biomed J [Internet]. 2017;40 (5):295–9.
51. Jadoul P, Kitajima M, Donnez O, Squifflet J, Donnez J. Surgical treatment of ovarian endometriomas: state of the art? Fertil Steril [Internet]. 2012;98(3):556–63.
52. Jacobson TZ, Barlow DH, Koninckx PR, Olive D, Farquhar C. Laparoscopic surgery for subfertility associated with endometriosis. Cochrane Database Syst Rev. 2002;4:CD001398.
53. Vercellini P, Fedele L, Aimi G, De Giorgi O, Consonni D, Crosignani PG. Reproductive performance, pain recurrence and disease re- lapse after conservative surgical treatment for endometriosis: the predictive value of the current classification system. Hum Reprod. 2006;21:2679–85.
54. Hart RJ, Hickey M, Maouris P, Buckett W. Excisional surgery versus ablative surgery for ovarian endometriomata. Cochrane Database Syst Rev. 2008;2:CD004992.
55. Practice Committees of the American Society for Reproductive Medicine and Society for Assisted Reproductive Technology. Intracytoplasmic sperm injection (ICSI) for non-male factor infertility: a committee opinion. Fertil Steril. 2012;98(6):1395–9.

56. ESHRE Guideline. Management of women with endometriosis. Hum Reprod. 2014;29 (3):400–12.
57. Duffy JMN, Arambage K, Correa FJS, Olive D, Farquhar C, Garry R, et al. Laparoscopic surgery for endometriosis. Cochrane Database Syst Rev. 2014;4:CD011031.
58. Adamson GD, Pasta DJ. Endometriosis fertility index: the new, validated endometriosis staging system. Fertil Steril. 2010;94(5):1609–15.
59. Jaafar SH, Sallam HN, Arici A, Garcia-Velasco JA, Abou-Setta AM. Long-term GnRH agonist therapy before in vitro fertilization (IVF) for improving fertility outcomes in women with endometriosis. Cochrane Database Syst Rev. 2019;1:CD013240. https://doi.org/10.1002/14651858.CD013240.
60. Sallam HN, Garcia-Velasco JA, Dias S, Arici A. Long-term pituitary down-regulation before in vitro fertilization (IVF) for women with endometriosis. Cochrane Database Syst Rev [Internet]. 2006;(1):CD004635.
61. Llarena NC, Falcone T, Flyckt RL. Fertility preservation in women with endometriosis. Clin Med Insight Reprod Health. 2019;13:1179558119873386. https://doi.org/10.1177/1179558119873386.
62. Adamyan LV, Dementyeva VO, Asaturova AV. New technique in reproductive surgery: one-step surgical procedure for ovarian function activation (first clinical observation). Akusherstvo i Ginekologiya/Obstet Gynecol. 2019;3:147–51. https://doi.org/10.18565/aig.2019.3.147-151. (in Russian)
63. Kawamura K, Cheng Y, Suzuki N, et al. Hippo signaling disruption and Akt stimulation of ovarian follicles for infertility treatment. Proc Natl Acad Sci U S A. 2013;110(43):17474–9. https://doi.org/10.1073/pnas.1312830110.
64. Senapati S, Sammel MD, Morse C, Barnhart KT. Impact of endometriosis on in vitro fertilization outcomes: an evaluation of the Society for Assisted Reproductive Technologies Database. Fertil Steril. 2016;106(1):164–171.e1. https://doi.org/10.1016/j.fertnstert.2016.03.037.
65. Somigliana E, Infantino M, Benedetti F, Arnoldi M, Calanna G, Ragni G. The presence of ovarian endometriomas is associated with a reduced responsiveness to gonadotropins. Fertil Steril. 2006;86:192–6.
66. Esinler I, Bozdag G, Arikan I, Demir B, Yarali H. Endometrioma ≤3 cm in diameter per se does not affect ovarian reserve in intracy- toplasmic sperm injection cycles. Gynecol Obstet Investig. 2012;74:261–4.
67. Hamdan M, Dunselman G, Li TC, Cheong Y. The impact of endometrioma on IVF/ICSI outcomes: a systematic review and meta- analysis. Hum Reprod Update. 2015;21:809–25.
68. Hong SB, Lee NR, Kim SK, Kim H, Jee BC, Suh CS, et al. In vitro fertilization outcomes in women with surgery induced diminished ovarian reserve after endometrioma operation: comparison with diminished ovarian reserve without ovarian surgery. Obstet Gynecol Sci. 2017;60:63–8.
69. Benschop L, Farquhar C, van der Poel N, Heineman MJ. Interventions for women with endometrioma prior to assisted reproductive technology. Cochrane Database Syst Rev. 2010;11:CD008571.
70. ETIC Endometriosis Treatment Italian Club. When more is not better: 10 'don'ts' in endometriosis management. An ETIC* position statement. Hum Reprod Open. 2019;2019(3)::hoz009. https://doi.org/10.1093/hropen/hoz009.
71. Vercellini P, Somigliana E, Vigano P, De Matteis S, Barbara G, Fedele L. The effect of second-line surgery on reproductive performance of women with recurrent endometriosis: a systematic review. Acta Obstet Gynecol Scand. 2009;88:1074–82.
72. Park H, Kim CH, Kim EY, Moon JW, Kim SH, Chae HD, et al. Effect of second-line surgery on in vitro fertilization outcome in infer- tile women with ovarian endometrioma recurrence after primary conservative surgery for moderate to severe endometriosis. Obstet Gynecol Sci. 2015;58:481–6.
73. Dunselman GA, Vermeulen N, Becker C, Calhaz-Jorge C, D'Hooghe T, De Bie B, et al. ESHRE guideline: management of women with endometriosis. Hum Reprod. 2014;29:400–12.

74. Adamyan LV, Starodubtseva N, Borisova A, et al. Direct mass spectrometry differentiation of ectopic and Eutopic endometrium in patients with endometriosis. J Minim Invasive Gynecol. 2018;25(3):426–33.
75. Kuznetsova MV, Pshenichnyuk EY, Burmenskaya OV, Asaturova AV, Trofimov DY, Adamyan LV. Study of gene expression in the eutopic endometrium of women with endometrioid cysts. Obstet Gynecol. 2017;8:93–102.
76. Adamyan LV, Osipova AA, Aznaurova YB, Sonova MM, Petrov IV, Suntsova MV, Buzdin AA. Analysis of gene expression and activation of signalling pathways in eutopic and ectopic endometrium of patients with external genital endometriosis. Vopr Ginekol Akus Perinatol (Gynecology, Obstetrics and Perinatology). 2019;18(1):6–10.

# ART and Endometriosis: Problems and Solutions

11

Iñaki González-Foruria and Pedro N. Barri Ragué

## 11.1 Introduction

Endometriosis is a benign gynaecological disease characterized by the presence of endometrial tissue outside the uterine cavity, primarily on the pelvic peritoneum and ovaries. The most common clinical features of endometriosis are dysmenorrhea, chronic pelvic pain, pain during intercourse, and infertility. However, the clinical symptoms do not always correlate with the extent of the disease, and for this reason, the diagnosis of the disease is often delayed between 7 and 10 years.

The real prevalence of endometriosis is unknown. There are no published studies on representative samples of the general population. In general, it is difficult to compare estimates of prevalence because the previously published studies include women with different conditions, and are conducted in centres that apply different diagnostic criteria and exhibit different levels of clinical interest in endometriosis. However, and according to prevalence estimates, it is accepted that this inflammatory disorder may affect up to 10–15% of women of reproductive age, representing a major health issue.

This work was performed under the auspices of the *Càtedra d'Investigació en Obstetrícia i Ginecologia* of the Department of Obstetrics, Gynaecology and Reproductive Medicine, Hospital Universitari Dexeus, Universitat Autònoma de Barcelona.

I. González-Foruria (✉) · P. N. Barri Ragué (✉)
Dexeus Mujer, Department of Reproductive Medicine, Dexeus University Hospital, Barcelona, Spain
e-mail: inagon@dexeus.com; PERBAR@dexeus.com

## 11.2    Relationship Between Endometriosis and Infertility

Establishing a causal relationship between endometriosis and infertility is based in many aspects. First of all, epidemiological data suggest such a link. In infertile women, previous studies show that the prevalence of endometriosis demonstrated by laparoscopy increases at least up to 30% [1]. More specifically, in normo-ovulatory women, with normospermic partners and at least 1 year of infertility, laparoscopy will show endometriosis findings in 47% of such patients [2]. In the same line, interesting research showed that patients with surgically confirmed endometriosis present lower chances of spontaneous conception than women with unexplained infertility (36% vs. 55%; $P < 0.05$) [3].

Secondly, and from a biological point of view, several rationales could explain a causal link between endometriosis and infertility. Although for ethical reasons, no experiments have looked for such association in humans, the nonhuman primate model of the baboon has been an excellent opportunity to demonstrate endometriosis-associated infertility [4]. Chronic inflammatory changes and increased oxidative stress present in the peritoneal fluid of patients with endometriosis may affect egg quality, folliculogenesis, luteal function, and more importantly, impair the sperm–oocyte interaction [5, 6]. Besides, the distortion of the normal anatomy of the ovaries and fallopian tubes due to fibrosis could hinder the tubo-ovarian functionality. And finally, an altered endometrial receptivity, endogenous cell production of estrogens with progesterone resistance, and dysperistalsis of the myometrium may negatively affect conception [5].

Finally, and in order to further reinforce such association, there is evidence that demonstrates that removing the potential cause may reduce the effect. In this regard, several publications have shown an increase in the chances of spontaneous conception after surgical removal of pelvic lesions in infertile women [7].

## 11.3    ART and Endometriosis

Endometriosis has become an important indication of in vitro fertilization (IVF) worldwide. In the United States in 2015, endometriosis was diagnosed in 8% of women who underwent IVF. In the United Kingdom in 2014, the diagnosis of endometriosis was made in 6% of the patients receiving IVF [8, 9]. In our Reproductive Medicine Department, at Dexeus University Hospital, a total of 13.6% of the IVF cycles performed during 2019 presented endometriosis as their main factor. Most of our patients were not previously operated for endometriosis and diagnosis was based upon a thorough transvaginal scan during common infertility work-up.

It is noteworthy that the golden standard for diagnosis of endometriosis is still the surgical removal and anatomopathological evaluation of the lesions. Nevertheless, nowadays, most patients who decide to pursue IVF have not been previously operated to rule out the presence of endometriotic lesions. In fact, most of the diagnoses are performed by means of imaging techniques, such as transvaginal ultrasound or magnetic resonance imaging, as they have shown a high accuracy in the endometriosis assessment [10]. In this regard, many cases of infertility of unknown origin could present an underlying endometriosis that has not been diagnosed, so the real prevalence of endometriosis in IVF cycles may be underestimated. It is, therefore, needless to remark the relevance and magnitude of the issue in assisted reproduction units worldwide.

## 11.4   IVF Results in Endometriosis

Although it has been a matter of debate for many years, the most recent publications on the topic demonstrate that, in general terms, patients with endometriosis have similar ART outcomes to those women without the disease. Although live birth rates are comparable, higher cancellation rates and a lower number of oocytes in patients with endometriosis have been published [11, 12]. Nevertheless, different authors claim that women with the most severe forms of the disease (e.g., stages III and IV according to the American Society of Reproductive Medicine [13]) present worse outcomes compared to patients with milder stages of the disease [14, 15].

Following the current knowledge that the higher the number of eggs obtained, the higher the cumulative live birth rates [16], it makes it hard to understand how previous studies have not found lower live birth rates when endometriosis patients tend to get fewer eggs than controls. Actually, most studies have not taken into account all embryos generated (either fresh or frozen) or were run in the era where the embryo-freezing was not so efficient as it is today. Therefore, they may have properly not analyzed cumulative live birth rates. For this reason, it is still a non-resolved question whether endometriosis negatively affects cumulative live birth rates.

With respect to the best ovarian stimulation protocol in endometriosis patients, it was for many years believed, that a long-term pituitary downregulation before IVF enhanced the chances of pregnancy by fourfold [17]. Nevertheless, after the analysis made by more recent studies, it seems that agonists and antagonists work equally in terms of pregnancy rates [18, 19], and there is rising concern regarding the real benefit of ultra-long agonist downregulation [20].

## 11.5   Endometrioma and ART

Ovarian endometrioma is probably the most known of the endometriosis phenotypes, as it is easily recognized by means of imaging techniques. Present in 17–44% of patients with endometriosis, the endometrioma management represents a challenge in the infertility approach [21]. Nowadays, it is commonly accepted that endometrioma surgery will negatively affect ovarian reserve [11, 22]. Surgical insults will not only decrease ovarian reserve markers [such as anti-müllerian hormone (AMH) and antral follicle count (AFC)] but will also reduce the number of oocytes obtained after ovarian stimulation in the operated gonads. It has to be highlighted that previous reports demonstrate a 2.4% risk of premature ovarian failure in surgeries with bilateral endometrioma removal [23].

There is still a current long-lasting debate on who is responsible for the lower AMH values found in patients with endometrioma: is it the endometrioma per se or is it the negative iatrogenic impact of surgery over the ovary? [24, 25]. Most authors agree that the main reason for such a decrease in ovarian reserve comes from previous ovarian surgeries, and not from the fact of presenting and endometrioma. Nevertheless, recent studies suggest that even with the same age and AMH levels, patients with endometrioma obtain less oocytes after ovarian stimulation for IVF and require higher doses of gonadotropins [26] (González-Foruria et al., in press). These findings suggest that patients with endometrioma present a lower ovarian sensitivity index than controls.

Despite the lack of randomized control trials, there is a common belief that laparoscopic treatment of endometrioma will enhance the chances of spontaneous pregnancy during the first months after surgery [21]. In these cases, pregnancy rates have been reported from 30% to 67%. On the other hand, it should be stressed that endometrioma removal before IVF is not going to increase clinical pregnancy rates compared to expectant management, but operated patients will require more days of stimulations, higher doses of gonadotropins and less oocytes will be obtained [23].

Taking into account the aforementioned information, the management of infertile patients with endometrioma has shifted in recent years from a surgical approach in most of the cases to a more conservative strategy [27]. In vitro fertilization will shorten the time to live birth, offering maximal chances of conception with extremely low complication rates. In this regard, ovarian stimulation and oocyte retrieval have both shown to be safe in patients with endometrioma. Data on the risks of infection, endometriosis pain, and disease progression are reassuring according to retrospective cohort studies [28, 29].

In the supposed cases of infertile patients with large endometriomas, previous surgeries, low ovarian reserve, or other comorbidities, the idea of a new surgical procedure is not recommended at all. Endometrioma drainage and sclerotherapy before ovarian stimulation and egg retrieval could represent an alternative for such cases, allowing the infertility specialist to gain technical access to the potential mature follicles of the affected ovaries [30]. The risk of infection and rapid recurrence of the endometrioma have to be taken into account before performing such procedure.

Finally, during oocyte retrieval, efforts should be taken in order to avoid going through the endometrioma. The endometriotic content is toxic for the oocyte, compromising blastulation and implantation rates, although fertilization rates are maintained.

## 11.6   Deep Infiltrating Endometriosis (DIE) and ART

The presence of DIE in IVF cycles is probably underrepresented in the literature. Actually, in the common infertility work-up performed before general IVF practice, DIE is not looked for, even if it is suspected for clinical data. Such overlook is the result of two situations. The first one is that in non-expert hands, DIE is not easy to find despite the use of transvaginal ultrasound. Secondly, despite presenting DIE most infertility specialists will not change the management of the patient. Nevertheless, we believe that it is of utmost importance to suspect and diagnose endometriosis, and specially DIE, in infertile patients before undergoing IVF. Although in most cases of infertile patients suffering from DIE, the decision to pursue IVF, the protocol, and the gonadotropin type and doses will remain unchanged, there are some relevant aspects that are worth evaluating before starting ART, so individual assessment of each case is mandatory. The first one, and probably the most important, is the clinics of the patient. Some of these women will suffer from unbearable dysmenorrhea or chronic pelvic pain that is not well tolerated with common analgesics. Others will complain of deep dyspareunia, dysuria, or cyclic dyschezia. To our understanding, there are few indications of surgery before ART in the endometriosis patient. However, unbearable pain leading to a bad quality of life is probably the main one. A thorough anamnesis questioning the patient about pain scores, history of past use of oral contraceptive pills for dysmenorrhea, or absenteeism from school or work for menstrual pain should lead the specialist to suspect endometriosis [31]. Afterwards, a meticulous physical exploration and imaging techniques should be carried out in order to reach the diagnosis. The second aspect to be taken into account before proceeding to ART is to discard those DIE locations that could compromise important structures such as the bowel (especially the rectum/sigmoid colon) or the ureter with potentially severe or even lethal complications. Although intestinal involvement of DIE is frequent (37% reported in some series), bowel occlusion due to an endometriotic implant is an extremely rare event. Severe ureteral endometriosis has been described in 4.6% of patients presenting DIE, most of them without renal consequences. Therefore, hydronephrosis and renal function loss are also rare complications of this disease [32]. No ART should be started in the presence of lesions that may potentially cause the aforementioned complications, and surgery should be previously considered. Lastly, surgery for endometriosis has been proposed by some authors as a potential treatment to overcome repeated implantation failure, though quality evidence on the topic is lacking.

Regarding IVF outcomes in DIE patients, it has been reported that patients with the most severe forms of the disease, present lower chances of pregnancy than milder stages [12, 14, 15]. The reasons for such negative impact are not completely understood, although inflammation will probably play a crucial role in pregnancy achievement. In this line, and with the aim of replacing embryos in a more natural endometrium far from the supraphysiological estradiol levels achieved during ovarian stimulation, some authors have proposed an elective freeze-all strategy. Today, in the era of embryo vitrification, the results of frozen–thawed embryo transfer are reassuring, so such a strategy should not be overlooked. Unfortunately, there are only a few retrospective series that have analyzed the question and the results are promising, suggesting better outcomes in terms of ongoing pregnancy rates following deferred frozen–thawed embryo transfer than with the fresh approach [33]. Prospective randomized controlled trials are needed to provide a definitive answer to whether we should continue transferring in the fresh cycle, or shift towards a deferred frozen–thawed embryo transfer approach in endometriosis patients. Interestingly, as not all endometriosis patients are the same, future research should be also directed towards identifying which patients may benefit from such a strategy. In freeze-all protocols for IVF, patients with endometriosis under antagonist protocol should be triggered with GnRH agonists, as their pain and discomfort is significantly reduced in comparison to classical hCG trigger [29].

Finally, apart from the marked increased risk of placenta previa in these patients (OR: 3.03; 95% CI 1.50–6.13) [34], it must be borne in mind that uncommon but potentially life-threatening acute complications from DIE in the pregnant women may arise, such as spontaneous hemoperitoneum, bowel perforation, and uterine rupture.

## 11.7    Adenomyosis and ART

Adenomyosis is considered a disease of the endomyometrial junction defined by the presence of heterotopic endometrial glands and stroma within the myometrium. As this condition frequently coexists with other forms of endometriosis, there is rising concern regarding the negative impact of adenomyosis in fertility and also in ART outcomes. The diagnosis of adenomyosis in the infertile women relies on imaging techniques without histologic verification, therefore leading to certain shortcomings. The present absence of strict image criteria and image classification of the extent of adenomyosis creates great heterogeneity among studies. Besides, the coexistence with different endometriosis phenotypes makes it even harder to draw valid conclusions on the outcomes of ART. Unfortunately, the quality of the studies that have analyzed the impact of adenomyosis in IVF cycles is poor, and the heterogeneity in the inclusion criteria is high. Notwithstanding, most studies point in the same direction, showing that either alone or in coexistence with endometriosis, IVF outcomes are clearly impaired in the presence of adenomyosis [35, 36]. Evidence is lacking regarding possible therapeutic options that could improve ART outcomes. A positive effect of long pituitary downregulation with GnRH agonists (for 3–6 months before implantation) has been suggested, though the number of patients analyzed is scanty to draw definitive conclusions. Cytoreductive surgery has been also proposed as an alternative for some patients in the absence of other medical options.

## 11.8   Which Is the Best Approach to the Infertile Endometriosis Patient Requiring IVF?

Although the heterogeneity of the infertile patient with endometriosis is enormous, and each case should be individualized, we provide a therapeutic algorithm for the management of these patients taking into account the more relevant aspects regarding their prognosis.

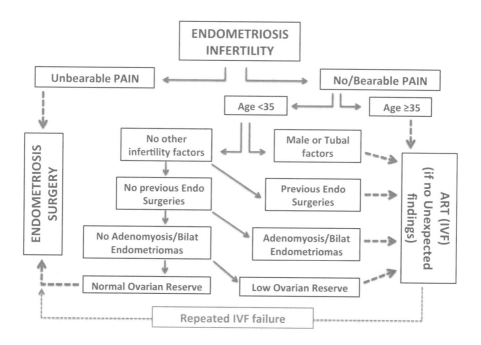

## 11.9   Egg Reception in Endometriosis

The negative influence of endometriosis on ovarian reserve and the quality of the obtained eggs seems evident. However, lower implantation rates raise the question of whether this finding is only the consequence of lower number and poorer quality of embryos, or whether it also reflects compromised endometrial receptivity. Egg donation programmes provide a unique model to investigate reproductive outcomes in these patients, as factors affecting the oocytes are excluded, especially if cycles using sibling oocytes derived from the same donor are analyzed. These studies, performed a few years ago, demonstrated reduced implantation rates in non-endometriotic patients who received oocytes from donors with endometriosis, whereas in recipients with endometriosis, healthy donated oocytes will contribute to a pregnancy with similar chances as in women without the disease [37]. The issue remains unclosed, as it is not clear whether previous endometrial priming protocols, such as GnRH agonists, given to endometriotic recipients, may have positively affected implantation. Although some research have analyzed egg donation outcomes in patients with adenomyosis [38], most studies did not account for the coexistence of adenomyosis following the current diagnostic imaging criteria, so further research is needed to give a definitive answer to this question.

## 11.10 Fertility Preservation in Endometriosis

During the last years, abundant bulk of evidence has demonstrated the detrimental effects of surgery for ovarian endometriomas over the ovarian reserve. During this time, indications for surgery have shrunk. Besides, biological and epidemiological findings make us believe that endometriosis patients will present lower chances of natural conception. Following such rationales, fertility preservation may be considered as an option for the endometriosis patient, not yet infertile. Nowadays, oocyte vitrification has become the most efficient fertility preservation procedure, no longer being considered experimental. Recently, Cobo et al. have presented a large cohort of endometriosis patients (1044 women) who decided to bank their oocytes [39]. The first striking data of this study is the high rate of women coming back to thaw their eggs (43%), when most studies in non-endometriotic patients have shown rates <10%. Besides, it is also noteworthy that the mean time between freezing and thawing is just 1.5 years. In this regard, as already recognized by the authors in the discussion, some of these patients were already infertile and decided to freeze their oocytes before an elective surgery that could impair their ovarian reserve. The second relevant finding of this milestone study is the high rate of success associated with the technique (46% of live birth rate per thawing procedure). Besides, among women who failed to become pregnant using their frozen eggs and decided to perform a new ovarian stimulation for IVF, 39% achieved a pregnancy. In the future, research will have to focus on how to identify which endometriosis patients will benefit from freezing their eggs. Data from Cobo et al. seem very reassuring, and although more studies are needed to consolidate their results, infertile specialists must be aware of the possibility of fertility preservation in endometriosis.

**Key Points**
- Endometriosis represents one of the main IVF indications worldwide.
- In general terms, IVF resulting in endometriosis are comparable to those in patients without the disease.
- May be impaired in patients with the most severe forms of the disease.
- There is no clear benefit of any ovarian stimulation protocol for IVF.
- Ovarian reserve is damaged after endometrioma surgery, and IVF results after surgery are not improved. Therefore, infertile patients with endometrioma should proceed with IVF to maximize their chances of conception.
- Ovarian stimulation and egg retrieval are safe procedures in terms of disease progression and pain.

- No ART should be started in the presence of lesions that may potentially cause severe complications, such as bowel occlusion or renal hydronephrosis due to extrinsic ureteral compression.
- Adenomyosis compromises IVF results, and there is no clear treatment to overcome such impairment.
- Egg donation presents comparable outcomes in recipients with and without endometriosis.
- Oocyte freezing as a fertility preservation technique has demonstrated to be a safe and efficient procedure and should be considered in the endometriosis patient.

# References

1. D'Hooghe TM, et al. Endometriosis and subfertility: is the relationship resolved? Semin Reprod Med. 2003;21(2):243–54.
2. Meuleman C, et al. High prevalence of endometriosis in infertile women with normal ovulation and normospermic partners. Fertil Steril. 2009;92(1):68–74.
3. Akande VA, et al. Differences in time to natural conception between women with unexplained infertility and infertile women with minor endometriosis. Hum Reprod. 2004;19(1):96–103.
4. D'Hooghe TM, et al. Nonhuman primate models for translational research in endometriosis. Reprod Sci. 2009;16(2):152–61.
5. de Ziegler D, Borghese B, Chapron C. Endometriosis and infertility: pathophysiology and management. Lancet. 2010;376(9742):730–8.
6. Gonzalez-Foruria I, et al. Dysregulation of the ADAM17/Notch signalling pathways in endometriosis: from oxidative stress to fibrosis. Mol Hum Reprod. 2017;23(7):488–99.
7. Duffy JM, et al. Laparoscopic surgery for endometriosis. Cochrane Database Syst Rev. 2014;4: CD011031.
8. Human Fertilisation and Embryology Authority. Fertility treatment 2014—Trends and figures. London 2016, 2016.
9. Centers for Disease Control and Prevention, American Society for Reproductive Medicine, Society for Assisted Reproductive Technology. 2015 Assisted reproductive technology national summary report. 2017. Atlanta, 2017.
10. Guerriero S, et al. Transvaginal ultrasound vs magnetic resonance imaging for diagnosing deep infiltrating endometriosis: systematic review and meta-analysis. Ultrasound Obstet Gynecol. 2018;51(5):586–95.
11. Hamdan M, et al. The impact of endometrioma on IVF/ICSI outcomes: a systematic review and meta-analysis. Hum Reprod Update. 2015;21(6):809–25.
12. Hamdan M, et al. Influence of endometriosis on assisted reproductive technology outcomes: a systematic review and meta-analysis. Obstet Gynecol. 2015;125(1):79–88.
13. Revised American Society for Reproductive Medicine classification of endometriosis: 1996. Fertil Steril. 1997;67(5):817–21.
14. Oppenheimer A, et al. Pregnancy rate after first intra cytoplasmic sperm injection- in vitro fertilisation cycle in patients with endometrioma with or without deep infiltrating endometriosis. Int J Fertil Steril. 2013;7(3):207–16.
15. Ballester M, et al. Deep infiltrating endometriosis is a determinant factor of cumulative pregnancy rate after intracytoplasmic sperm injection/in vitro fertilization cycles in patients with endometriomas. Fertil Steril. 2012;97(2):367–72.
16. Polyzos NP, et al. Cumulative live birth rates according to the number of oocytes retrieved after the first ovarian stimulation for in vitro fertilization/intracytoplasmic sperm injection: a multicenter multinational analysis including approximately 15,000 women. Fertil Steril. 2018;110 (4):661–70. e1

17. Sallam HN, et al. Long-term pituitary down-regulation before in vitro fertilization (IVF) for women with endometriosis. Cochrane Database Syst Rev. 2006;1:CD004635.
18. Drakopoulos P, et al. Does the type of GnRH analogue used, affect live birth rates in women with endometriosis undergoing IVF/ICSI treatment, according to the rAFS stage? Gynecol Endocrinol. 2018;34(10):884–9.
19. Rodriguez-Purata J, et al. Endometriosis and IVF: are agonists really better? Analysis of 1180 cycles with the propensity score matching. Gynecol Endocrinol. 2013;29(9):859–62.
20. Georgiou EX, et al. Long-term GnRH agonist therapy before in vitro fertilisation (IVF) for improving fertility outcomes in women with endometriosis. Cochrane Database Syst Rev. 2019;2019(11):CD013240.
21. Chapron C, et al. Management of ovarian endometriomas. Hum Reprod Update. 2002;8(6):591–7.
22. Rossi AC, Prefumo F. The effects of surgery for endometriosis on pregnancy outcomes following in vitro fertilization and embryo transfer: a systematic review and meta-analysis. Arch Gynecol Obstet. 2016;294(3):647–55.
23. Garcia-Velasco JA, Somigliana E. Management of endometriomas in women requiring IVF: to touch or not to touch. Hum Reprod. 2009;24(3):496–501.
24. Muzii L, et al. Antimullerian hormone is reduced in the presence of ovarian endometriomas: a systematic review and meta-analysis. Fertil Steril. 2018;110(5):932–40. e1
25. Somigliana E, et al. Surgical excision of endometriomas and ovarian reserve: a systematic review on serum antimullerian hormone level modifications. Fertil Steril. 2012;98(6):1531–8.
26. Bourdon M, et al. Endometriosis and ART: a prior history of surgery for OMA is associated with a poor ovarian response to hyperstimulation. PLoS One. 2018;13(8):e0202399.
27. Barri PN, et al. Endometriosis-associated infertility: surgery and IVF, a comprehensive therapeutic approach. Reprod BioMed Online. 2010;21(2):179–85.
28. Villette C, et al. Risks of tubo-ovarian abscess in cases of endometrioma and assisted reproductive technologies are both under- and overreported. Fertil Steril. 2016;106(2):410–5.
29. Santulli P, et al. Endometriosis-related infertility: assisted reproductive technology has no adverse impact on pain or quality-of-life scores. Fertil Steril. 2016;105(4):978–87. e4
30. Cohen A, Almog B, Tulandi T. Sclerotherapy in the management of ovarian endometrioma: systematic review and meta-analysis. Fertil Steril. 2017;108(1):117–24. e5
31. Chapron C, et al. Questioning patients about their adolescent history can identify markers associated with deep infiltrating endometriosis. Fertil Steril. 2011;95(3):877–81.
32. Chapron C, et al. Deeply infiltrating endometriosis: pathogenetic implications of the anatomical distribution. Hum Reprod. 2006;21(7):1839–45.
33. Bourdon M, et al. The deferred embryo transfer strategy improves cumulative pregnancy rates in endometriosis-related infertility: A retrospective matched cohort study. PLoS One. 2018;13(4):e0194800.
34. Zullo F, et al. Endometriosis and obstetrics complications: a systematic review and meta-analysis. Fertil Steril. 2017;108(4):667–72. e5
35. Sharma S, et al. Does presence of adenomyosis affect reproductive outcome in IVF cycles? A retrospective analysis of 973 patients. Reprod BioMed Online. 2019;38(1):13–21.
36. Vercellini P, et al. Uterine adenomyosis and in vitro fertilization outcome: a systematic review and meta-analysis. Hum Reprod. 2014;29(5):964–77.
37. Hauzman EE, Garcia-Velasco JA, Pellicer A. Oocyte donation and endometriosis: what are the lessons? Semin Reprod Med. 2013;31(2):173–7.
38. Martinez-Conejero JA, et al. Adenomyosis does not affect implantation, but is associated with miscarriage in patients undergoing oocyte donation. Fertil Steril. 2011;96(4):943–50.
39. Cobo A, et al. Oocyte vitrification for fertility preservation in women with endometriosis: an observational study. Fertil Steril. 2020;113(4):836–44.

# Morphokinetics in Embryos from Patients with Endometriosis

**12**

Paolo Giovanni Artini, Elena Pisacreta, Susanna Cappellini, and Elena Carletti

## 12.1 Introduction

Endometriosis is one of the most common and controversial women-related diseases. It is defined as the presence and cyclical growth of functional endometrial tissue (glands and stroma) outside the uterus, commonly occurring on the ovaries and peritoneum [1]. Endometriosis could be considered as a heterotopy in which the ectopic endometrium is influenced by estrogenic stimuli and cyclically proliferates, and becomes a secretory tissue and breaks down, as well as the endometrial mucosa [2].

It is a chronic condition that affects women in reproductive age and the main symptoms of the disease are chronic pelvic pain, dysmenorrhea, dyspareunia, and infertility (endometriosis is diagnosed in 25–40% of infertile women) [3, 4].

It is estimated that between 10% and 15% [5, 6] of women of reproductive age have endometriosis but it is difficult to estimate accurately because the diagnosis is still made with laparoscopic view of the lesions and their biopsy [7, 8]. In fact, nowadays, there is no serum markers or imaging techniques that are able to replace the role of surgical visualization and histological analyses [9].

P. G. Artini (✉)
Division of Gynecology and Obstetrics, Department of Experimental and Clinical Medicine, University of Pisa, Pisa, Italy

Fertility IVF&Unit "Pina De Luca" Casa di Cura Privata San Rossore, Pisa, Italy
e-mail: paolo.artini@unipi.it

E. Pisacreta · S. Cappellini
Division of Gynecology and Obstetrics, Department of Experimental and Clinical Medicine, University of Pisa, Pisa, Italy

E. Carletti
Fertility IVF&Unit "Pina De Luca" Casa di Cura Privata San Rossore, Pisa, Italy

Several studies demonstrate the central role of inflammation and oxidative stress (with *ROS* production) [10–12] even if it is unknown whether inflammation predisposes to, or result from, endometriosis. Inflammation is involved at various levels [13] (peritoneal fluid, follicular fluid, uterine endometrium) demonstrated by the elevation in cytokines, prostaglandins, and chemokines. This inflamed microenvironment affects the reproductive potential of women with endometriosis, at first harming oocytes quality and embryos development [14, 15].

For the severe stages of endometriosis, infertility can be explained by the anatomic changes in the pelvic cavity. Instead of the minimal and mild stages, it is much more difficult to explain the reason for infertility.

### 12.1.1 Oocyte Quality

After the pick-up, oocytes should be evaluated analyzing their morphological assessment [16]. It is based on the aspects of:

- Granulosa cells.
- Oocyte–corona–cumulus complex (OCCC).
- Oocyte cytoplasm (color, shape, and graininess).

The evaluation of these parameters provides information about the stage of development:

- Oocyte with an expanded radiating corona surrounded by cumulus cells is classified as mature.
- Oocyte with expanded cumulus cells, slightly compact corona radiate, and uneven color is classified as intermediate.
- Oocyte with dense compact cumulus and adherent compact layer of corona is classified as immature.
- Oocyte with dark and irregularly expanded cumulus with few cells and dark corona is classified as post-mature.

In this way, the embryologist has an idea of the subsequent developmental ability of the driving embryo and excludes from insemination oocytes of bad quality (these assessments are particularly important for oocytes candidates for IVF-ET) [17].

However, this classification has important limits because, at the time of retrieval, the oocyte is hidden by the cumulus mass and there is only a poor correlation between the morphology of OCCCs and the outcome of fertilization, cleavage, and clinical pregnancy rates.

The evaluation of real oocyte maturity is possible only after denudation of the oocyte from its cumulus and corona cells; the best condition for this is during *Intracytoplasmatic sperm injection* (ICSI) because it provides the removal of OCCC.

In this way, oocyte is classified into:

- Oocyte in metaphase II stage (MII): the first polar body (PB) is visible in the perivitelline space (PVS). This is the best oocyte to be fertilized.
- Oocyte in metaphase I stage (MI): it has neither a visible germinal vesicle (GV) nor PB. A good percentage of oocytes in this stage reaches MII (in vitro maturation).
- Oocyte in prophase I stage: the oocyte has a visible GV. Oocytes in this stage are immature and the fertilization percentage is very poor.

At the pick-up, 60–70% of the oocytes have at least one morphological abnormality (cytoplasmic or extracytoplasmic). As cytoplasmic abnormalities, we describe: changes in cytoplasm color (more dark), presence of granulation (central or diffuse), presence of vacuoles, and presence of refractive bodies. On contrary, extracytoplasmic abnormalities include: alterations in zona pellucida (thicker and/or more dark), alterations of PVS (enlarged and/or with graininess), and PB anomalies (fragmented or abnormally shaped) [18].

## 12.1.2 Embryo Quality

After fertilization, oocytes are cultured in incubators with an environment designed to reproduce the human fallopian tube. Seventeen hours after fertilization, embryologists should find out how many oocytes have really fertilized and they should be able to correlate the features observed at the optical microscope with the implantation potential of each particular embryo.

A normally fertilized oocyte (zygote) should have:

- Two pronuclei (PN) which represent sperm and oocyte genetic information.
- Two PBs which come from oocyte meiotic division.

If an oocyte is seen to have more or less than two PNs or two PBs, it means that it has not or abnormally fertilized and it is separated from other zygotes.

Over the years, parameters for the evaluation of the zygote, embryo, and blastocyst have been variously proposed and lacked a widespread comprehension. This is why in 2011 *The Istanbul consensus workshop on embryo assessment* [19] proposed parameters to be universally accepted.

*The Consensus* shows important parameters such as the number of cells in the embryo specific-per day (embryos division either too slow or too fast could be damaged in chromosomic information), their aspect at microscope (size, the degree of fragmentation, the symmetry of the cells, the presence of multinucleation, and the compaction status). Cleavage stage embryos range from the two-cell stage (2C, early cleavage check) to the compacted morula composed of 8–16 cells (day 4).

According to *The Consensus* the classification that should be used is:

- Embryo grade I: <10% fragmentation, stage-specific cell size, no multinucleation (Fig. 12.1).

**Fig. 12.1** Embryo grade I

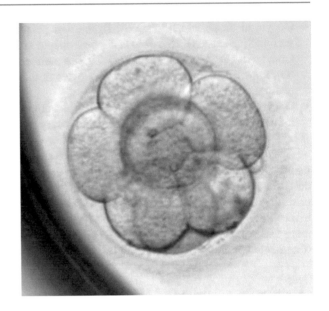

**Fig. 12.2** Embryo grade III

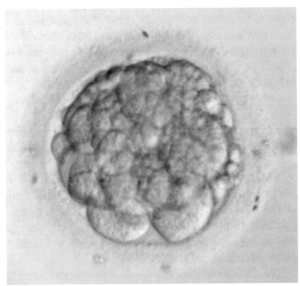

- Embryo grade II: 10–25% fragmentation, stage-specific cell size for the majority of cells, no evidence of multinucleation.
- Embryo grade III: >25% fragmentation, cell size not stage-specific, evidence of multinucleation (Fig. 12.2).

## 12.1.3 Advantages in Technology

Most attempts to analyze embryo quality in endometriosis have been so far established on static observation of their morphology. Advances in technology and their application to embryology have led to the development of time-lapse incubators, which allow to keep the embryos in culture and have continuous morphokinetic data (sequential images) thanks to the presence of small cameras inside. Cameras collect images in real time with a very high frequency (intervals of 5–10 min) and, for each embryo in culture, make a movie that reproduces each stage of embryonic development. This allows the embryologists to have information about early stages of embryonic development and to detect changes that generally occur at extremely slow speeds so that they are normally imperceptible to direct observation. Moreover, this system allows to control embryos development without extracting them from the incubator and so without exposing embryos to external changes (temperature, pH, gas), which would adversely affect their development.

Normally, the choice of the embryo to be transferred is made by traditional observation only on a morphological basis of the embryo; on the contrary, the time-lapse system allows to make a choice based on division kinetics (timing of embryos division) and early morphokinetic changes in real time.

## 12.1.4 Endometriosis Versus Control (Tubal Factor Infertility)

Our study has been structured in order to evaluate if endometriosis affects oocyte and embryo development, by comparing parameters such as the number of aspirated follicles, number of retrieved oocytes, number of normal or abnormal zygote (respectively 2PN and 1PN/3PN), and number of embryos grade I, II, and III.

At these parameters, we also added the evaluation of morphokinetics of endometriotic embryos compared to control embryos.

We have included nine patients with endometriosis (stage II or III according to the classification of *The American Society of Reproductive Medicine*, ASRM) and nine patients with tubal factor infertility. For our study, we ruled out patients with female-associated infertility factors and/or male infertility in order to make our sample the most homogeneous and to avoid selection bias.

All patients underwent a complete clinical history and physical examination, biochemical analyses, transvaginal ultrasonography, and only in vitro fertilization cycles (IVF).

We followed embryo dynamic development using a time-lapse system with *Genea Biomedx* incubator. It has six incubation chambers and each one is designed to contain embryos of a single patient and has a dedicated camera. Each chamber is organized in 16 micro-wells, in each of which there is a single embryo to be monitored. This allows the incubator to contain and control six patients for a total of 96 embryos simultaneously.

From the comparison of endometriosis and control group, we find out that (Table 12.1):

**Table 12.1** Parameters in endometriosis and control group, with t-test

|                                       | Endometriosis group Average ± SD | Control group Average ± SD |
| ------------------------------------- | -------------------------------- | -------------------------- |
| Number of patients                    | 9                                | 9                          |
| Age                                   | 35.33 ± 2.74                     | 34.20 ± 2.59               |
| Retrieved oocytes                     | 7.22 ± 4.12                      | 10.20 ± 5.36               |
| Retrieved oocytes/aspirated follicles | 69.9%                            | 83.6%                      |
| Zygotes 2PN                           | 4.22 ± 3.53                      | 6.40 ± 4.04                |
| Oocytes in MII                        | 6.44 ± 4.25                      | 8.80 ± 6.06                |
| Evolutive embryo                      | 2.78 ± 2.28                      | 4.20 ± 2.39                |
| Embryo grade I                        | 0.33 ± 0.50                      | 1.80 ± 1.30                |
| Embryo grade III                      | 0.78 ± 0.97                      | 0.00 ± 0.00                |

- Age: there is no significant difference in the mean age of endometriosis and control group.
- Number of retrieved oocytes: significantly lower in women with endometriosis than in the control group ($7.22 \pm 4.12$ vs. $10.20 \pm 5.36$ with $p = 0.01$); furthermore, for this parameter, it is interesting to note the different percentage between the two groups in relation to the percentage of retrieved oocyte based on aspirated follicles (69.9% in endometriosis vs. 83.6% in control patients).
- Number of zygotes 2PN: significantly lower in women with endometriosis than in the control group ($4.22 \pm 3.53$ vs. $6.40 \pm 4.04$, with $p = 0.01$).
- Number of oocytes in MII: significant difference between endometriosis and control group (respectively $6.44 \pm 4.25$ and $8.80 \pm 6.06$ with $p = 0.04$).
- Number of embryo grade III: there is a significant difference between the number of embryo grade III in endometriosis and control group (respectively $0.78 \pm 0.97$ vs. $0.00 \pm 0.00$ with $p = 0.04$).

## 12.1.5 Morphokinetics of Endometriotic Embryo at Time-Lapse

Time-lapse system allows us to evaluate morphokinetics of the embryo early development. It seems that there is a trend of lag in the endometriosis group for the fusion of PNs and for the first division. In fact, from our analysis, it turned out that for syngamy of the 2 PNs, it needs $28 \pm 3.7$ h in endometriosis group, versus $27 \pm 3.7$ h in the control group; also for the first division, it needs $31 \pm 4.8$ h in endometriosis group versus $30 \pm 3.8$ h in the control group. These data are not statistically significant yet (probably our sample is too small) but they could demonstrate that the endometriosis has an influence even at these levels of the reproduction process.

| Dynamic system | Endometriosis group Average ± SD | Control group Average ± SD |
|---|---|---|
| Time for syngamy | 28 ± 3.7 h | 27 ± 3.7 h |
| Time for first division | 31 ± 4.8 h | 30 ± 3.8 h |

With the dynamic method, it was also possible to evaluate embryo multinucleation and fragmentation at first division (2C stage). Multinucleation and fragmentation are two negative factors that directly correlate with poor embryo quality (*The Consensus* defines embryo grade even on % of fragmentation and presence of multinucleation) and they are regarded as important parameters for the embryologist to select embryos to be transferred. Our results show how multinucleation and fragmentation are much more present in endometriotic evolutive embryos than in the control group (from a total of 25 evolutive embryo in the endometriosis group and 38 in the control group):

- As concerns multinucleation, it is present in about 20% of endometriotic evolutive embryos versus 5% in the control group.
- As concerns fragmentation at 2C stage, only 26% of the embryo from the control group presents more than 25% of fragmentation; on contrary, in endometriosis group, 36% of evolutive embryo presents more than 25% of fragmentation (Fig. 12.3).

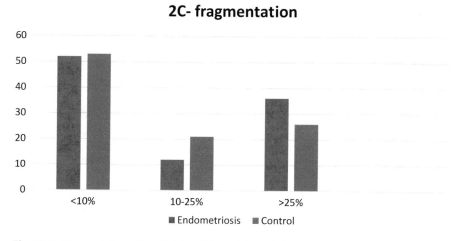

**Fig. 12.3** Fragmentation at first division (2C stage) in evolutive embryos of the endometriosis and control group

## 12.1.6 Final Consideration

Endometriosis seems to affect many aspects of female reproductive function by interfering with the endocrine system (hypothalamic–pituitary–ovarian axis), oocyte and embryo quality, uterine receptivity at the time of implantation, and with the probability of implanting itself [13]. Probably, the inflamed microenvironment in which endometriotic oocytes develop deeply affects oocyte and embryo fertility potential not only in the number of retrieved oocytes, zygotes 2PNs, embryos grade but also in the division kinetics (differences in multinucleation, fragmentation of endometriotic embryos). With the dynamic system (time-lapse) we wanted to observe any anomalies (in addition to the morphological ones) linked to the morphokinetics of the embryos of women affected by endometriosis in early stages of their development in order to better understand the effects of endometriosis condition on embryo quality. Certainly, there is a trend for endometriotic embryos to have both the time required for syngamy and the time required for first cell division, approximately 1 h longer than the control. This result, even if it should be confirmed in a larger sample, could be another proof of how endometriosis influences women reproductive ability at 360°.

## References

1. Giudice LC, Kao LC. Endometriosis. Lancet. 2004;364(9447):1789–99.
2. Pescetto G, Cecco LD, Pecorari D, Ragni N. Ginecologia e ostetricia, vol. 1. Roma: SEU; 2017. p. 15–32.
3. Xu B, et al. Oocyte quality is decreased in women with minimal or mild endometriosis. Sci Rep. 2015;5:10779.
4. The Practice Committee of the American Society for Reproductive Medicine. Endometriosis and infertility: a committee opinion. Fertil Steril. 2012;98(3):591–8.
5. Augoulea A, et al. Pathogenesis of endometriosis: the role of genetics, inflammation and oxidative stress. Arch Gynecol Obstet. 2012;286(1):99–103.
6. Singh N, et al. Effect of endometriosis on implantation rates when compared to tubal factor in fresh non donor in vitro fertilization cycles. J Hum Reprod Sci. 2014;7(2):143–7.
7. Hadfield R, et al. Delay in the diagnosis of endometriosis: a survey of women from the USA and the UK. Hum Reprod. 1996;11(4):878–80.
8. Eskenazi B, Warner ML. Epidemiology of endometriosis. Obstet Gynecol Clin N Am. 1997;24(2):235–58.
9. Kavoussi SK, et al. New paradigms in the diagnosis and management of endometriosis. Curr Opin Obstet Gynecol. 2016;28(4):267–76.
10. Da Broi MG, et al. Increased concentration of 8-hydroxy-2′-deoxyguanosine in follicular fluid of infertile women with endometriosis. Cell Tissue Res. 2016;366(1):231–42.
11. Malvezzi H, et al. Peritoneal fluid of women with endometriosis reduces SOD1 in bovine oocytes in vitro maturation. Cell Tissue Res. 2018;372(3):621–8.
12. Jianini B, et al. Peritoneal fluid from infertile women with minimal/mild endometriosis compromises the meiotic spindle of metaphase II bovine oocytes: a pilot study. Reprod Sci. 2017;24(9):1304–11.
13. Stilley JA, Birt JA, Sharpe-Timms KL. Cellular and molecular basis for endometriosis-associated infertility. Cell Tissue Res. 2012;349(3):849–62.

14. Brosens I. Endometriosis and the outcome of in vitro fertilization. Fertil Steril. 2004;81 (5):1198–200.
15. Olivennes F. Results of IVF in women with endometriosis. J Gynecol Obstet Biol Reprod (Paris). 2003;32(8 Pt 2):S45–7.
16. Veeck LL. An atlas of human gametes and conceptuses: an illustrated reference for assisted reproductive technology. London: Taylor & Francis; 1999.
17. Sathananthan AH, Gunasheela S. Human oocyte and embryo assessment for ART. In: Human preimplantation embryo selection. Boca Raton, FL: CRC Press; 2007. p. 1–14.
18. Rienzi LF, Ubaldi F. Oocyte retrieval and selection. In: Texbook of assisted reproductive technologies. Laboratory and clinical perspective. Boca Raton, FL: CRC Press; 2009. p. 85–101.
19. Balaban B. The Istanbul consensus workshop on embryo assessment: proceedings of an expert meeting. Hum Reprod. 2011;26(6):1270–83.

# Endometriosis and Cancer: Prevention and Diagnosis

**13**

Silvia Vannuccini, Sara Clemenza, and Felice Petraglia

## 13.1 Introduction

Endometriosis is a benign gynecological condition, affecting approximately 5–15% of all women [1]. It is an inflammatory and estrogen-dependent disease characterized by the presence of endometrial tissue outside the uterus, mainly on pelvic organs but also in extragenital sites [2]. Although endometriosis causes chronic symptoms, such as dysmenorrhea, dyspareunia, pelvic pain, and infertility, affecting widely quality of life, it is considered a benign disease of reproductive age women [3]. However, it has been estimated that 0.3–0.8% of endometriosis cases are complicated by neoplasia, mainly ovarian cancer [4]. Several common pathways linking endometriosis and ovarian cancer have been elucidated, including the involvement of some cytokines, oxidative stress, and a hyper-estrogenic hormonal milieu [5].

Ovarian cancer is the most fatal gynecological cancer. More than 90% of ovarian tumors have an epithelial origin, whereas the others arise from germ cells or granulosa-theca cells. Among epithelial tumors, about 60–70% are serous (further subdivided in high (90–95%) and low grade (5–10%)), 5% are mucinous, and 15% are either endometrioid and clear cell [6]. The link between endometriosis and ovarian cancer was first identified in 1925 by Sampson, who proposed the criteria

S. Vannuccini (✉)
Obstetrics and Gynecology, Department of Experimental and Clinical Biomedical Sciences, Careggi University Hospital, University of Florence, Florence, Italy

Department of Molecular and Developmental Medicine, University of Siena, Siena, Italy
e-mail: silvia.vannuccini@unifi.it

S. Clemenza
Obstetrics and Gynecology, Department of Experimental and Clinical Biomedical Sciences, Careggi University Hospital, University of Florence, Florence, Italy

F. Petraglia
Obstetrics and Gynecology Division, University of Florence, Firenze, Italy

© International Society of Gynecological Endocrinology 2021
A. R. Genazzani et al. (eds.), *Endometriosis Pathogenesis, Clinical Impact and Management*, ISGE Series, https://doi.org/10.1007/978-3-030-57866-4_13

to identify this condition: evidence of endometriosis close to the tumor, demonstration of cancer arising within ovarian endometriosis and finding of endometrial stroma surrounding characteristic epithelial glands [7]. Then, in 1953, a morphological continuity between benign and malignant epithelium in endometriosis was demonstrated [8].

Endometriosis-associated ovarian cancer (EAOC) represents a heterogeneous group of different types of cancer including clear cell carcinoma, endometrioid carcinoma, and seromucinous borderline tumor, arising in case of coexistent endometriosis. In fact, EAOC is described as an ovarian cancer having both cancer cells and endometriosis in the same ovary, presence of cancer in one ovary and endometriosis in the second ovary or presence of ovarian cancer and pelvic endometriosis [9]. Indeed, endometriosis is associated with a significantly increased risk of clear-cell ovarian cancer (CCOC) and endometrioid ovarian cancer (ENOC) [10]. In fact, in women with ENOC a 26.3% positive history for endometriosis was shown and 21.1% in CCOC [11]. Furthermore, co-existent endometriosis in ovarian cancer lesions was found in 40.6% of CCOC cases and 23.1% of ENOC [12].

There are molecular and biological evidences to suggest an association between endometriosis and ovarian cancer, such as self-sufficiency in proliferation signals, resistance to apoptosis, tissue invasiveness, the dominance of certain cytokines, oxidative stress, hyper-estrogenic hormonal milieu, and genetic mutations [13].

However, considering the discrepancy between the low prevalence of ENOC and CCOC and the high prevalence of endometriosis, the hypothesis that endometriosis represents an exclusive premalignant condition remains to be demonstrated. Although it appears to be an association between endometriosis and EAOC, endometriosis is not considered a premalignant lesion and a specific screening is not recommended, if endometriosis is not atypical. Moreover, there are no conclusive data indicating that prophylactic removal of all endometriosis lesions reduces the risk of EAOC [14].

## 13.2  Epidemiology and Risk Factors

The lifetime risk of ovarian cancer ranges from 1.4% in the general population to about 1.9% in women with endometriosis [14]. The prevalence of epithelial ovarian cancer in women with endometriosis is reported to be 2–17.0%, whereas the prevalence of endometriosis in those who are diagnosed with epithelial ovarian cancer ranges from 3.4% to 52.6%, suggesting a huge difference among studies [15]. This is due to the high heterogeneity of analyzed populations; in addition, the different criteria used to diagnose endometriosis could account for the great difference in the incidence rate of ovarian cancer among those women.

CCOC and ENOC are the most frequent histotypes associated with endometriosis [14]. A large collaborative effort by the Ovarian Cancer Association Consortium (OCAC) reported that endometriosis increases the risk of CCOC by threefold, and the risk of low-grade serous and ENOC subtypes by twofold, whereas mucinous and high-grade serous cancers appear not to be associated with the disease

[10]. Furthermore, a recent Finnish study on the association between cancer and endometriosis phenotypes showed that the risk is the highest among women with ovarian endometriosis (OMA), especially for ENOC (incidence ratio 4.72 (2.75–7.56)) and CCOC (incidence ratio 10.1 (5.50–16.9)), occurring 5–10 years after the index surgery. On the contrary, no increased risk of cancer has been found among women with peritoneal and deep infiltrating endometriosis [16].

Women with EAOC tend to be younger (45–50 years old) and with lower-grade and lower stage of cancer than the general population of women with ovarian cancer. The possible explanation for this evidence is that benign symptomatic disease leads to an increased number of examinations and imaging assessments, which in turn may lead to an earlier diagnosis of ovarian cancer [17]. Furthermore, the frequency of endometriosis in postmenopausal women is lower than in the premenopausal ones, but the risk of ovarian cancer is higher. Increasing age is one of the major risk factors associated with EAOC [18]. Women aged >50 years with endometriosis had significantly higher risk of EOC than age-matched women without endometriosis or those affected by endometriosis but younger than 30 years [19].

Endometriosis shares many risk factors with epithelial ovarian cancer, such as early menarche, late menopause, infertility, and nulliparity [20, 21]. On the contrary, multiple pregnancies, prolonged lactation, and late menarche are protective [22].

Prolonged oral contraceptives (OC) use is associated with a significant reduction in the risk of developing an endometrioma, maybe for ovulation inhibition. It was shown that the use of OCs for >10 years may cause a reduction in ovarian cancer risk among women with endometriosis [20]. Unfortunately, data on the effect of OC specifically on EAOC is still not available and the protective effect of OC seems to be relevant only if prolonged use and in fertile age.

## 13.3 Pathogenesis

The molecular mechanisms underlying the malignant transformation of endometriosis remains controversial and yet to be clarified. However, the pathogenetic hypothesis in which endometriosis is considered an early stage of a multi-step development process that culminates in ovarian cancer seems plausible.

It was suggested that atypical endometriosis may represent the intermediate step in neoplastic progression. Atypical endometriosis is characterized by abnormal cells that exhibit an increased nuclear/cytoplasmic ratio, mild hyperchromasia, mild to moderate pleomorphism, and presents with an intermediate proliferation activity between typical endometriosis and ovarian cancer [23]. Therefore, several authors indicate only atypical endometriosis as a premalignant lesion [9]. Although the pathogenetic transformation from endometriosis to ovarian cancer is not fully understood, it seems related to the cooperation of multiple factors such as genetic aberrations, oxidative stress, inflammation, and hyperestrogenism [24] (Fig. 13.1).

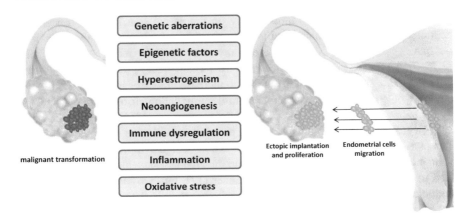

**Fig. 13.1** Endometriosis and cancer: pathogenetic mechanisms involved in malignant transformation

## 13.3.1 Genetic Aberrations

Endometriosis is characterized by abnormal cell proliferation and alterations in apoptosis [25]. Histologically benign endometriosis may harbor genetic abnormalities that predispose for malignant transformation [26, 27]. Mutations of ARID1A, a tumor suppressor gene, have been demonstrated in atypical endometriosis, indicating that ARID1A is involved in the early stages of EAOC development [28]. In fact, inactivating ARID1A mutations are the most common molecular genetic alteration reported in CCOC and ENOC. These mutations result in loss of expression of the protein encoded by ARID1A (BAF250a), which normally suppresses cellular proliferation through a p53-dependent transcription regulation of several tumor suppressors. Loss of protein expression of the ARID1A tumor suppressor gene has been demonstrated also in endometriosis adjacent to clear cell tumor samples and atypical endometriosis suggesting an important role in the malignant transformation of endometriosis [29].

Also, PIK3CA mutations are common in CCOC. The phosphoinositide 3-kinase (PI3K) pathway plays a key role in cell proliferation and survival in response to growth factors, hormones, and cytokines. It seems to play an important role in the pathogenesis of CCOC; PIK3CA mutations were found in the coexisting endometriotic epithelium adjacent to the clear cell carcinoma and atypical endometriosis, suggesting a possible role in tumor development in endometriosis [30].

A number of studies have showed that mutation of the *PTEN* tumor suppressor gene occurs frequently in endometriosis cysts, CCOC, and ENOC [31]. Microsatellite instability (MSI) leading to the functional inactivation of the PTEN gene was also found in atypical endometriosis, suggesting that endometriosis and atypical endometriosis may act as precursor lesions that have the potential to progress into EAOC [32].

KRAS is one of the most frequently mutated genes in ovarian endometriotic epithelium. Mutations in the KRAS gene lead to constitutive activation of the KRAS-BRAF-MEK-MAPK signaling pathway, influencing cellular proliferation, apoptosis, adhesion, and migratory capacity. Molecular alterations of KRAS are also found in ENOC [33].

## 13.3.2 Epigenetic Factors

Several studies have demonstrated common epigenetic alterations between endometriosis and ovarian cancer [24]. The epigenetic modifications involved in EAOC include DNA methylation, histone modifications, and noncoding miRNAs. For example, hypermethylation of the promoter region of hMLH1, which has a role in DNA mismatch repair, and of Runt-related transcription factor (RUNX3) has been found in endometriosis and seems to be associated with its malignant evolution [34]. Furthermore, endometriotic stromal cells contain widespread epigenetic defects that alter gene expression, drive inflammation, inducing, ovarian epithelial cells proliferation, through estrogen-mediated pathways [27].

## 13.3.3 Inflammation and Hyperestrogenism

Inflammation is a typical feature of endometriosis, as the presence of ectopic tissue in the peritoneal cavity is associated with overproduction of prostaglandins, cytokines, and chemokines [2]. The pelvic fluid from women with endometriosis has increased concentrations of macrophages and inflammatory cytokines, particularly TNF-$\alpha$, IL-$\beta$, and IL-6 [35]. These same cytokines have been reported at significantly higher concentrations in cell cultures of epithelial ovarian cancer [36]. The chronic inflammatory pelvic environment of women with endometriosis may facilitate the transformation of a normal endometrial cell into a malignant cell.

Moreover, endometriosis is characterized by increased estrogen sensitivity and progesterone resistance, responsible for aberrant mechanisms setting up positive feedback for cell proliferation [37]. Hyperestrogenism can result in cellular proliferation through the stimulation of cytokine production and prostaglandin E2 (PGE2), which in turn stimulates the activity of aromatase, resulting in a positive feedback loop in favor of hyperestrogenism [38]. This highly proliferative microenvironment in endometrioma results in an enhanced level of reparative activity, with a higher chance for DNA damage and mutations [2]. This is supported also by the observation that extra-ovarian localizations of endometriosis very rarely become malignant. Therefore, a specific role seems to be played by the ovarian microenvironment where endometriotic stromal cells have a number of epigenetic defects that alter gene expression and induce a progesterone-resistant and intensely inflammatory environment, driven by estrogen via estrogen receptor-$\beta$ [2]. The increased estrogenic action in the stroma causes inflammation and survival signals for epithelial cell proliferation. The hyperestrogenism in the ovary also induces direct genotoxic effect on

DNA, causing accumulation of additional mutations and malignant transformation of ovarian epithelial cells.

### 13.3.4 Oxidative Stress

Oxidative stress refers to the physiological imbalance between the presence of reactive oxygen species (ROS) and the ability of the body to eradicate them. ROS may cause DNA damage, playing an important role in the initiation and promotion phases of carcinogenesis. Endometriosis is characterized by repeated bleeding into the cyst cavity during the menstrual cycle [39]. Blood cells in the extravascular space tend to lyse quickly and heme is released. Free heme promotes oxidative damage and formation of ROS, which split the heme ring and release redox-active free iron. Free iron is a strong oxidant and contributes to the production of ROS. Persistent exposure to highly concentrated free iron may contribute to ovarian carcinogenesis due to the production of oxidative stress and, consequently, DNA damage, mutations, and genomic instability [40].

### 13.3.5 Angiogenesis and Immune Dysregulation

Neoangiogenesis is necessary for the development and sustenance of endometriotic lesions as the peritoneal environment is poorly vascularized compared to the endometrial eutopic tissue [41]. Also, tumoral cells require newly formed vessels to obtain oxygen and nutrients necessary for continuous proliferation [42]. Vascular endothelial growth factor (VEGF) has been detected in high concentrations in peritoneal fluid of women with endometriosis and it is also the most potent and specific angiogenic factors that should contribute to EAOC. Other proangiogenic factors, such as hepatocyte growth factor (HGF), erythropoietin, angiogenin, macrophage migration inhibitory factor, neutrophil-activating factor, and TNF-α, have been found at increased concentrations in the peritoneal fluid of patients with endometriosis. It could be of interest to know whether concentrations are further elevated in EAOC [43].

Impaired cellular and humoral immunity have been reported in endometriotic tissue, causing a reduced clearance of refluxed endometrial cells [44]. The hypothesis that an altered immune response plays a role in the pathogenesis of the disease is supported by the increased incidence of autoimmune disorders in patients with endometriosis. The main immune alterations concern natural killer cells, macrophages, neutrophils, humoral immunity, cytokines, and growth factors. Cytokines and growth factors seem to promote implantation, growth (inducing proliferation and angiogenesis), and invasion of the ectopic endometrium. Alteration in the complement pathway and humoral immunity was also identified in EAOC [45]. Furthermore, in vitro results indicated that the KRAS and PTEN/PI3K pathways increased complement gene expression. These data seem to suggest that immunological factors are significantly involved in the pathogenesis of endometriosis and EAOC.

## 13.4  Diagnosis of Endometriosis-Associated Ovarian Cancer (EAOC)

Transvaginal ultrasound (TVUS) represents the first imaging approach in the evaluation of endometriosis and ovarian cancer. The accuracy of an expert's subjective assessment (pattern recognition) of the gray-scale and Doppler ultrasound image is very high. The "typical" endometrioma is a unilocular or multilocular (one to four locules) cystic formation with thick, regular walls and homogeneous hypoechoic content, defined "ground glass," without septa, with little peripheral vascularization and absence of central vascularization [46–48]. However, "atypical" ultrasound features have been described in up to 35% of endometrioid cysts, indicating that sometimes diagnosis might be challenging. Atypical endometriomas differ from the classic endometrioma for the presence of inhomogeneous echogenicity, internal septations, irregular margins, calcification, papillary projection without flow [49] (Fig.13.2).

Furthermore, the ultrasonographic characteristics of endometriomas may differ according to pre- or postmenopausal status. In older women, multilocular cysts and

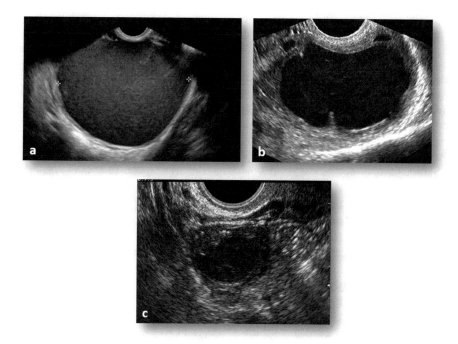

**Fig. 13.2** "Typical endometrioma" (**a**) and "atypical endometrioma" (**b, c**)

cysts with papillations and other solid components become more common, whereas ground glass echogenicity of cyst fluid becomes less common compared to endometriomas observed in younger women. This explains the poorer diagnostic performance of ultrasound for endometriomas in premenopausal women aged more than 40 years compared with younger women [50]. On one side, papillary projections and solid components increase the risk of malignancy but may occur also in endometriomas, especially in older women. Therefore, in postmenopausal women, the appearances of an atypical endometrioma should be examined very carefully as there is a significant risk of malignancy in such lesions in this age group [49].

The diagnostic ultrasound-based discrimination of benign versus malignant ovarian masses arising in endometrioid cysts might rely on the same ultrasound features characterizing malignant versus benign nature in all ovarian masses. Therefore, suspicious ultrasound features of malignant transformation in endometrioid cyst are [51]:

- Presence of solid tissue.
- Papillary projections: the number of papillae is significant, as in ovarian cancer the number of papillae is often greater than 3.
- Vascularization of the solid component at color Doppler evaluation.
- Ascites.
- Heterogeneous cystic content due to the presence of solid parts, necrosis, and hemorrhage in the mass.

The rapid growth of an endometrioma in perimenopause or during hormonal treatment in fertile age, the presence of solid vascularized components and the change in echogenicity are signs of suspicious ovarian lesion [52]. In addition, whereas in premenopausal women the majority of solid components observed within ovarian endometriomas are retracted blood clots, in older women this finding should be interpreted as a suspect [53]. The most reliable predictors of the development of ovarian cancer among women with ovarian endometrioma are advancing age (>45 years) and mass size (>8 cm) [18, 54]. Overall, in a large series of endometrioma surgically treated, the incidence of EAOC was 0.14%; in the majority of those cases, the patient's age was above 40 years and papillary projections were found into the cysts during the preoperative assessment [55].

Furthermore, it has been shown that ENOC, if arising from endometriosis, have specific ultrasound characteristics. While EOCs are usually large, unilateral, multilocular-solid, or solid tumors, if developing from endometriosis, they are more often unilateral cysts with papillary projections and no ascites [56]. However, there is still a lack of evidences showing the specific sonographic features of atypical endometriomas versus those observed in premalignant endometriomas, which will degenerate into cancer.

Regarding useful biomarkers for the diagnosis of EAOC, nowadays there are no additional tools to identify patients with endometriosis at elevated risk of ovarian cancer. CA125 is the most widely used serum biomarker in ovarian cancer.

However, it is rarely helpful in the differential diagnosis between a benign endometrioma and a malignant ovarian mass, as CA125 levels are often raised in women with endometriosis [57]. A future prospect seems to be the use of miRNAs as biomarkers for early detection and diagnosis of EAOC [58]. MicroRNAs (miRNAs) are single-stranded non-coding small RNA molecules that regulate gene expression by inhibiting mRNA translation or by facilitating cleavage of the target mRNA. They are frequently dysregulated in human cancers, including EAOC. miRNAs are exceptionally stable and can be readily and reliably detected in the systematic circulation raising the possibility of using blood-based miRNA assays to develop novel biomarkers for cancer detection, diagnosis, and prognosis. Overexpression of serum miR-16, 21, and 191 has been reported in EAOC and may be promising biomarkers of endometriosis-to-EAOC progression [59].

## 13.5 Clinical Implications of Endometriosis as a Risk Factor for Cancer

The discussion about the management of women with endometriosis, considering the increased risk for cancer, is mainly related to cases with ovarian localization in perimenopause, as for those in fertile age ovarian preservation and desire of pregnancy should be considered first [14]. No conclusive data are available on the effect of strict imaging surveillance versus surgical treatment (unilateral salpingo-oophorectomy or cystectomy/partial ovarian excision) on the mortality from EAOC in perimenopausal women with endometrioma. Some studies reported that endometrioma excision does not prevent the subsequent development of ovarian cancer [60]. On the contrary, in a case–control study, Rossing et al. indicated a protective effect of unilateral salpingo-oophorectomy for ovarian cancer in women with endometrioma, whereas cystectomy/partial ovarian excision did not reduce this risk [61]. Another case–control study showed that one-sided oophorectomy, i.e., extirpation of the affected ovary, as well as complete extirpation of all visible endometriosis, had a strong protective effect against ovarian cancer, even though it is unclear which histotypes are reduced [62].

It is well known that unilateral salpingo-oophorectomy results in a significant decrease in ovarian cancer risk, especially serous ovarian cancer. Thus, also the risk of overall ovarian cancer mortality is reduced by definition. However, this effect may be largely due to a decrease in the risk of death from high-grade serous carcinomas following salpingectomy, rather than from ENOC and CCOC following removal of ovaries with endometriomas. Therefore, it is still unknown whether surgical removal of ovaries with endometriomas is more effective than surveillance, in terms of reduced mortality from EAOC [14]. Because of a lack of conclusive evidence, there are no recommendations on the management of patients with endometriosis to reduce cancer risk. Moreover, as screening is not available for ovarian cancer, there is no clear management plan that would help to reduce a possible small increased risk [63]. Therefore, there needs to be a balance between women being fully informed about their condition (including related risks), with rationales for not encouraging unnecessary treatments.

Vercellini et al. proposed the removal of the affected ovary/ovaries plus bilateral salpingectomy in perimenopausal women with small (<5 cm), typical endometriomas, especially in cases of long-standing lesions. Otherwise, a strict surveillance, by serial TVUS scans, may be proposed; in case of modifications of sonographic features (cyst volume increase, presence of septa, papillary projections, mural nodules, or changes in vascularization) or suspicious rise in serum CA 125 and human epididymis protein 4 (HE4) levels, immediate surgery should be performed. Unfortunately, insufficient data are available on medical treatment (i.e., progestins) during surveillance and potential variation of EAOC risk when hormonal therapies are started during perimenopause. Thus, there is no rationale supporting the use of hormonal treatments after menopause, neither as a preventive nor as a therapeutic measure [14].

In women with a previous diagnosis of endometriosis, but without current evidence of endometriomas, there are no sufficient data to justify systematic risk-reducing salpingo-oophorectomy [64]. Regarding women who are diagnosed with atypical endometriosis, they should be counseled about the potential risk of recurrence and of possible small risk of progression to EAOC; in these patients, surgery could be considered.

The treatment should be personalized based on the patient's age, desire to bear children, family history, and type and characteristics of endometriomas. Moreover, the medical history of the patient must be considered because, especially when multiple and extensive abdominopelvic procedures have been performed, the operative risk may be increased to the point that sometimes the balance may be tipped toward expectant management.

## 13.6 Prognosis and Treatment of EAOC

Patients with EAOC are usually younger and had early-stage and low-grade disease compared to those without endometriosis. This, in turn, is related to the trend of better survival outcomes. The reason for early-stage diagnosis might be due to the signs and symptoms related to endometriosis that lead to frequent follow-ups; on the other hand, patients with no associated endometriosis may have had significant symptoms only when in later stages.

However, some studies did not find a better prognosis for ovarian cancer patients with previous or coexisting endometriosis, when the confounding effects of the stage are taken into account. In fact, women with endometriosis-associated ovarian cancer may receive an earlier diagnosis but, unfortunately, the longer time-span between diagnosis and death compared with women affected by ovarian cancer without endometriosis does not appear to result in a longer final survival [65]. Therefore, it remains to be determined whether endometriosis is a significant prognostic factor [15]. There is currently no substantiating evidence to support that women with

EAOC require different therapeutic options than those used in the treatment of all epithelial ovarian cancer.

Since there are no data to support a different type of treatment for these women, most are treated similarly to all epithelial ovarian cancers. As many of these women present early, they can be surgically staged, and receive the standard postoperative chemotherapy if disease is found outside the ovary.

## 13.7 Conclusion

Available data show a small increased risk of ovarian cancer in women with ovarian endometriosis, especially clear cell and endometrioid histotypes. On the contrary, those with peritoneal or deep endometriosis do not show a higher risk of malignancies. Atypical endometriosis is thought to be a precursor of ovarian cancer in the transformation from benign endometriosis to carcinoma. Since the evidences are limited and no screening for ovarian cancer is available, there are no recommendations on the management of patients with endometriosis to reduce cancer risk. Clinicians should inform women with endometriosis about their condition and related risks, without creating anxiety and encouraging unnecessary treatments. There is a theoretical rationale to believe that surgical and hormonal control of endometriosis may also decrease the risk of ovarian cancer. However, there are no data to date to support such a conclusion. Additional studies on the molecular progression of endometriosis to cancer are needed to identify which women are at higher risk for malignant transformation, in order to develop better prevention, screening, and treatment approaches.

## References

1. Zondervan KT, Becker CM, Missmer SA. Endometriosis. N Engl J Med. 2020;382:1244–56.
2. Bulun SE, Yilmaz BD, Sison C, Miyazaki K, Bernardi L, Liu S, Kohlmeier A, Yin P, Milad M, Wei J. Endometriosis. Endocr Rev. 2019b;40:1048–79.
3. Zondervan KT, Becker CM, Koga K, Missmer SA, Taylor RN, Viganò P. Endometriosis. Nat Rev Dis Primers. 2018 Jul 19;4(1):9.
4. Wei JJ, William J, Bulun S. Endometriosis and ovarian cancer: a review of clinical, pathologic, and molecular aspects. Int J Gynecol Pathol. 2011;30:553–68.
5. Ruderman R, Pavone ME. Ovarian cancer in endometriosis: an update on the clinical and molecular aspects. Minerva Ginecol. 2017;69:286–94.
6. Mok SC, Kwong J, Welch WR, Samimi G, Ozbun L, Bonome T, Birrer MJ, Berkowitz RS, Wong KK. Etiology and pathogenesis of epithelial ovarian cancer. Dis Markers. 2007;23:367–76.
7. Sampson JA. Endometrial carcinoma of the ovary arising in endometrial tissue in that organ. Arch Surg. 1925;10:1–72.
8. Scott RB. Malignant changes in endometriosis. Obstet Gynecol. 1953;2:283–9.
9. Grandi G, Toss A, Cortesi L, Botticelli L, Volpe A, Cagnacci A. The association between Endometriomas and ovarian Cancer: preventive effect of inhibiting ovulation and menstruation during reproductive life. Biomed Res Int. 2015;2015:751571.

10. Pearce CL, Templeman C, Rossing MA, Lee A, Near AM, Webb PM, Nagle CM, Doherty JA, Cushing-Haugen KL, Wicklund KG, et al. Association between endometriosis and risk of histological subtypes of ovarian cancer: a pooled analysis of case-control studies. Lancet Oncol. 2012;13:385–94.

11. Vercellini P, Parazzini F, Bolis G, Carinelli S, Dindelli M, Vendola N, Luchini L, Crosignani PG. Endometriosis and ovarian cancer. Am J Obstet Gynecol. 1993;169:181–2.

12. Jimbo H, Yoshikawa H, Onda T, Yasugi T, Sakamoto A, Taketani Y. Prevalence of ovarian endometriosis in epithelial ovarian cancer. Int J Gynaecol Obstet. 1997;59:245–50.

13. Dawson A, Fernandez ML, Anglesio M, Yong PJ, Carey MS. Endometriosis and endometriosis-associated cancers: new insights into the molecular mechanisms of ovarian cancer development. Ecancermedicalscience. 2018;12:803.

14. Vercellini P, Viganò P, Buggio L, Makieva S, Scarfone G, Cribiù FM, Parazzini F, Somigliana E. Perimenopausal management of ovarian endometriosis and associated cancer risk: when is medical or surgical treatment indicated? Best Pract Res Clin Obstet Gynaecol. 2018;51:151–68.

15. Heidemann LN, Hartwell D, Heidemann CH, Jochumsen KM. The relation between endometriosis and ovarian cancer - a review. Acta Obstet Gynecol Scand. 2014;93:20e31.

16. Saavalainen L, Lassus H, But A, Tiitinen A, Härkki P, Gissler M, Pukkala E, Heikinheimo O. Risk of gynecologic Cancer according to the type of endometriosis. Obstet Gynecol. 2018;131:1095–102.

17. Worley MJ, Welch WR, Berkowitz RS, Ng SW. Endometriosis-associated ovarian cancer: a review of pathogenesis. Int J Mol Sci. 2013;14:5367–79.

18. Kobayashi H, Sumimoto K, Kitanaka T, Yamada Y, Sado T, Sakata M, Yoshida S, Kawaguchi R, Kanayama S, Shigetomi H, Haruta S, Tsuji Y, Ueda S. Terao T ovarian endometrioma–risks factors of ovarian cancer development. Eur J Obstet Gynecol Reprod Biol. 2008;138:187–93.

19. Wang KC, Chang WH, Lee WL, Huang N, Huang HY, Yen MS, Guo CY, Wang PH. An increased risk of epithelial ovarian cancer in Taiwanese women with a new surgico-pathological diagnosis of endometriosis. BMC Cancer. 2014;14:831.

20. Modugno F, Ness RB, Allen GO, Schildkraut JM, Davis FG, Goodman MT. Oral 920 contraceptive use, reproductive history, and risk of epithelial ovarian cancer in women with 921 and without endometriosis. Am J Obstet Gynecol. 2004;191:733–40.

21. Stewart LM, Holman CD, Aboagye-Sarfo P, Finn JC, Preen DB. Hart R in vitro fertilization, endometriosis, nulliparity and ovarian cancer risk. Gynecol Oncol. 2013;128:260–4.

22. Torng PL. Clinical implication for endometriosis associated with ovarian cancer. Gynecol Minim Invasive Ther. 2017;6:152–6.

23. LaGrenade A, Silverberg SG. Ovarian tumors associated with atypical endometriosis. Case Reports Hum Pathol. 1988;19:1080–4.

24. Herreros-Villanueva M, Chen CC, Tsai EM, Er TK. Endometriosis-associated ovarian cancer: what have we learned so far? Clin Chim Acta. 2019;493:63–72.

25. Reis FM, Petraglia F, Taylor RN. Endometriosis: hormone regulation and clinical consequences of chemotaxis and apoptosis. Hum Reprod Update. 2013 Jul-Aug;19(4):406–18.

26. Anglesio MS, Papadopoulos N, Ayhan A, Nazeran TM, Noë M, Horlings HM, Lum A, Jones S, Senz J, Seckin T, Ho J, Wu RC, Lac V, Ogawa H, Tessier-Cloutier B, Alhassan R, Wang A, Wang Y, Cohen JD, Wong F, Hasanovic A, Orr N, Zhang M, Popoli M, McMahon W, Wood LD, Mattox A, Allaire C, Segars J, Williams C, Tomasetti C, Boyd N, Kinzler KW, Gilks CB, Diaz L, Wang TL, Vogelstein B, Yong PJ, Huntsman DG, Shih IM. Cancer-associated mutations in endometriosis without Cancer. N Engl J Med. 2017;376:1835–48.

27. Bulun SE, Wan Y, Matei D. Epithelial mutations in endometriosis: link to ovarian Cancer. Endocrinology. 2019a;160:626–38.

28. Ayhan A, Mao TL, Seckin T, Wu CH, Guan B, Ogawa H, et al. Loss of ARID1A expression is an early molecular event in tumor progression from ovarian endometriotic cyst to clear cell and endometrioid carcinoma. Int J Gynecol Cancer. 2012;22:1310–5.

29. Yamamoto S, Tsuda H, Takano M, Tamai S, Matsubara O. Loss of ARID1A protein expression occurs as an early event in ovarian clear-cell carcinoma development and frequently coexists with PIK3CA mutations. Mod Pathol. 2012;25:615–24.
30. Yamamoto S, Tsuda H, Takano M, Iwaya K, Tamai S, Matsubara O. PIK3CA mutation is an early event in the development of endometriosis-associated ovarian clear cell adenocarcinoma. J Pathol. 2011;225:189–94.
31. Smith IN, Briggs JM. Structural mutation analysis of PTEN and its genotype-phenotype correlations in endometriosis and Cancer. Proteins. 2016;84:1625–43.
32. Govatati S, Kodati VL, Deenadayal M, Chakravarty B, Shivaji S, Bhanoori M. Mutations in the PTEN tumor gene and risk of endometriosis: a case-control study. Hum Reprod. 2014;29:324–36.
33. Stewart CJ, Leung Y, Walsh MD, Walters RJ, Young JP, Buchanan DD. KRAS mutations in ovarian low-grade endometrioid adenocarcinoma: association with concurrent endometriosis. Hum Pathol. 2012;43:1177–83.
34. Ren F, Wang D, Jiang Y, Ren F. Epigenetic inactivation of hMLH1 in the malignant transformation of ovarian endometriosis. Arch Gynecol Obstet. 2012;285:215–21.
35. Hou Z, Sun L, Gao L, Liao L, Mao Y, Liu J. Cytokine array analysis of peritoneal fluid between women with endometriosis of different stages and those without endometriosis. Biomarkers. 2009;14:604–18.
36. Darai E, Detchev R, Hugol D, Quang NT. Serum and cyst fluid levels of interleukin (IL)-6, IL-8 and tumour necrosis factor-alpha in women with endometriomas and benign and malignant cystic ovarian tumours. Hum Reprod. 2003;18:1681–5.
37. Yilmaz BD, Bulun SE. Endometriosis and nuclear receptors. Hum Reprod Update. 2019;25:473–85.
38. Monsivais D, Dyson MT, Yin P, Coon JS, Navarro A, Feng G, Malpani SS, Ono M, Ercan CM, Wei JJ, Pavone ME, Su E, Bulun SE. ERβ- and prostaglandin E2-regulated pathways integrate cell proliferation via Ras-like and estrogen-regulated growth inhibitor in endometriosis. Mol Endocrinol. 2014;28:1304–15.
39. Scutiero G, Iannone P, Bernardi G, Bonaccorsi G, Spadaro S, Volta CA, Greco P, Nappi L. Oxidative stress and endometriosis: a systematic review of the literature. Oxidative Med Cell Longev. 2017;2017:7265238.
40. Kajiyama H, Suzuki S, Yoshihara M, Tamauchi S, Yoshikawa N, Niimi K, Shibata K, Kikkawa F. Endometriosis and cancer. Free Radic Biol Med. 2019;133:186–92.
41. Laschke MW, Giebels C, Menger MD. Vasculogenesis: a new piece of the endometriosis puzzle. Hum Reprod Update. 2011;17:628–36.
42. Králíčková M, Losan P, Vetvicka V. Endometriosis and cancer. Womens Health (Lond). 2014;10:591–7.
43. Laschke MW, Menger MD. Basic mechanisms of vascularization in endometriosis and their clinical implications. Hum Reprod Update. 2018;24:207–24.
44. Riccio LDGC, Santulli P, Marcellin L, Abrão MS, Batteux F, Chapron C. Immunology of endometriosis. Best Pract Res Clin Obstet Gynaecol. 2018;50:39–49.
45. Suryawanshi S, Huang X, Elishaev E, Budiu RA, Zhang L, Kim S, Donnellan N, Mantia-Smaldone G, Ma T, Tseng G, Lee T, Mansuria S, Edwards RP, Vlad AM. Complement pathway is frequently altered in endometriosis and endometriosis-associated ovarian cancer. Clin Cancer Res. 2014;20:6163–74.
46. Exacoustos C, Manganaro L, Zupi E. Imaging for the evaluation of endometriosis and adenomyosis. Best Pract Res Clin Obstet Gynaecol. 2014;28:655e81.
47. Guerriero S, Ajossa S, Mais V, et al. The diagnosis of endometriomas using colour Doppler energy imaging. Hum Reprod. 1998;6:1691–5.
48. Van Holsbeke C, Van Calster B, Guerriero S, Savelli L, Paladini D, Lissoni AA, Czekierdowski A, Fischerova D, Zhang J, Mestdagh G, Testa AC, Bourne T, Valentin L, Timmerman D. Endometriomas: their ultrasound characteristics. Ultrasound Obstet Gynecol. 2010;35:730–40.

49. Guerriero S, Condous G, van den Bosch T, Valentin L, Leone FP, Van Schoubroeck D, Exacoustos C, Installé AJ, Martins WP, Abrao MS, Hudelist G, Bazot M, Alcazar JL, Gonçalves MO, Pascual MA, Ajossa S, Savelli L, Dunham R, Reid S, Menakaya U, Bourne T, Ferrero S, Leon M, Bignardi T, Holland T, Jurkovic D, Benacerraf B, Osuga Y, Somigliana E, Timmerman D. Systematic approach to sonographic evaluation of the pelvis in women with suspected endometriosis, including terms, definitions and measurements: a consensus opinion from the International Deep Endometriosis Analysis (IDEA) group. Ultrasound Obstet Gynecol. 2016a;48:318–32.

50. Guerriero S, Van Calster B, Somigliana E, Ajossa S, Froyman W, De Cock B, Coosemans A, Fischerová D, Van Holsbeke C, Alcazar JL, Testa AC, Valentin L, Bourne T, Timmerman D. Age-related differences in the sonographic characteristics of endometriomas. Hum Reprod. 2016b;31:1723–31.

51. Testa AC, Timmerman D, Van Holsbeke C, Zannoni GF, Fransis S, Moerman P, Vellone V, Mascilini F, Licameli A, Ludovisi M, Di Legge A, Scambia G, Ferrandina G. Ovarian cancer arising in endometrioid cysts: ultrasound findings. Ultrasound Obstet Gynecol. 2011;38:99–106.

52. Nezhat FR, Apostol R, Nezhat C, Pejovic T. New insights in the pathophysiology of ovarian cancer and implications for screening and prevention. Am J Obstet Gynecol. 2015;213:262–7.

53. Tanase Y, Kawaguchi R, Takahama J, Kobayashi H. Factors that differentiate between endo-metriosis-associated ovarian Cancer and benign ovarian endometriosis with mural nodules. Magn Reson Med Sci. 2018;17:231–7.

54. He ZX, Shi HH, Fan QB, Zhu L, Leng JH, Sun DW, et al. Predictive factors of ovarian carcinoma for women with ovarian endometrioma aged 45 years and older in China. J Ovarian Res. 2017;10:45.

55. Kuo HH, Huang CY, Ueng SH, Huang KG, Lee CL, Yen CF. Unexpected epithelial ovarian cancers arising from presumed endometrioma: a 10-year retrospective analysis. Taiwan J Obstet Gynecol. 2017;56:55–61.

56. Moro F, Magoga G, Pasciuto T, Mascilini F, Moruzzi MC, Fischerova D, Savelli L, Giunchi S, Mancari R, Franchi D, Czekierdowski A, Froyman W, Verri D, Epstein E, Chiappa V, Guerriero S, Zannoni GF, Timmerman D, Scambia G, Valentin L, Testa AC. Imaging in gynecological disease (13): clinical and ultrasound characteristics of endometrioid ovarian cancer. Ultrasound Obstet Gynecol. 2018;52:535–43.

57. Dochez V, Caillon H, Vaucel E, Dimet J, Winer N, Ducarme G. Biomarkers and algorithms for diagnosis of ovarian cancer: CA125, HE4, RMI and ROMA, a review. J Ovarian Res. 2019;12:28.

58. Moga MA, Bălan A, Dimienescu OG, Burtea V, Dragomir RM, Anastasiu CV. Circulating miRNAs as biomarkers for endometriosis and endometriosis-related ovarian Cancer-an over-view. J Clin Med. 2019;8:735.

59. Suryawanshi S, Vlad AM, Lin HM, Mantia-Smaldone G, Laskey R, Lee M, Lin Y, Donnellan N, Klein-Patel M, Lee T, Mansuria S, Elishaev E, Budiu R, Edwards RP, Huang X. Plasma microRNAs as novel biomarkers for endometriosis and endometriosis-associated ovarian can-cer. Clin Cancer Res. 2013;19:1213–24.

60. Taniguchi F. New knowledge and insights about the malignant transformation of endometriosis. J Obstet Gynaecol Res. 2017;43:1093.

61. Rossing MA, Cushing-Haugen KL, Wicklund KG, Doherty JA, Weiss NS. Risk of epithelial ovarian cancer in relation to benign ovarian conditions and ovarian surgery. Cancer Causes Control. 2008;19:1357e64.

62. Melin AS, Lundholm C, Malki N, Swahn ML, Sparèn P, Bergqvist A. Hormonal and surgical treatments for endometriosis and risk of epithelial ovarian cancer. Acta Obstet Gynecol Scand. 2013;92:546e54.

63. National Institute for Health and Care Excellence. Endometriosis: diagnosis and management. NICE guideline NG73. September 2017. https://www.nice.org.uk/guidance/ng73/evidence/full-guideline-pdf-4550371315.

64. Wilbur MA, Shih IM, Segars JH, Fader AN. Cancer implications for patients with endometriosis. Semin Reprod Med. 2017;35:110–6.
65. Paik ES, Kim TJ, Choi CH, Kim BG, Bae DS, Lee JW. Clinical outcomes of patients with clear cell and endometrioid ovarian cancer arising from endometriosis. J Gynecol Oncol. 2018;29: e18.

# Medical Management of Endometriosis, Present and Future with Special Reference to MHT in the Patient Previously Diagnosed with Endometriosis

# 14

Tobie J. de Villiers

## 14.1   Introduction

The endometrium is the unique inner lining of the uterus that responds to the cyclical ovarian hormones estrogen and progesterone with the ultimate aim of providing a suitable implantation environment for the developing embryo. Endometriosis is defined as the presence of endometrial-like tissue outside the uterus that induces a chronic, inflammatory reaction [1]. Endometriosis is a chronic and incurable disease that causes pain and is associated with infertility. Adenomyosis is an associated condition where the endometrial tissue exists within and grows into the uterine myometrium. Adenomyosis will not be specifically addressed in this chapter. The aim of this chapter is to empower the reader with the options of hormonal treatment in endometriosis. Insight into the mechanism of actions, efficacy, and side-effect profile will enable the reader to individualize treatment to the best benefit of the victims of endometriosis.

Surgery will continue to be an important mode of treatment for endometriosis. In recent years, hormonal treatment has emerged as a major player in the management of endometriosis, either as solo therapy or as adjuvant therapy to surgery. This is not surprising as the behavior of endometrial tissue is modulated by hormones.

## 14.2   Prevalence of Endometriosis

The exact prevalence is unknown and may have a geographical variance, but estimates range from 2% to 10% of women of reproductive age, to 50% of infertile women [1]. A prospective study in 1991 of premenopausal women undergoing

T. J. de Villiers (✉)
Department of Gynaecology, Stellenbosch University and Mediclinic Panorama, Cape Town, South Africa
e-mail: tobie@iafrica.com

© International Society of Gynecological Endocrinology 2021
A. R. Genazzani et al. (eds.), *Endometriosis Pathogenesis, Clinical Impact and Management*, ISGE Series, https://doi.org/10.1007/978-3-030-57866-4_14

laparoscopy for different indications yielded the following percentage of histologically confirmed endometriosis: infertility (21%), sterilization (6%), and chronic pain (15%) [2].

## 14.3 Symptoms of Endometriosis

Pelvic pain is the most common symptom. It is classically described as being accentuated in the premenstrual period but maybe acyclic in character. Other pain-related symptoms are dysmenorrhea, dyspareunia, and pain with pelvic examination.

Many patients present with infertility. This may be the case even in the absence of ovarian-fimbrial involvement. Menometrorrhagia may be present. It should be noted that some patients may be asymptomatic.

## 14.4 Pathogenesis of Endometriosis

The exact pathogenesis of endometriosis remains unknown. The theory of retrograde menstruation as the cause of endometriosis dates back to 1924 [3]. It states that as the endometrial tissue breaks down, fragments travel up the fallopian tubes in a retrograde fashion into the peritoneal cavity. Successful implantation of endometriotic tissue probably requires additional cofactors such as an altered immune system, abnormal cytokine production, increased vascular supply, and increased cellular proliferation. Evidence in support of this theory include the higher volumes of refluxed menstrual blood seen in women with endometriosis and menstrual outflow obstruction. Other popular theories include coelomic metaplasia as well as angiogenic and lymphogenic spread of endometrial cells [4]. More recently, the genetic and epigenetic theory has been proposed to explain observations on different types of endometriosis as well as differences in biological behavior [5]. It proposes a set of genetic and epigenetic incidents transmitted at birth. Further development into typical simple endometriosis, cystic ovarian endometriosis or deep endometriosis lesions, then requires a series of additional transmissible genetic and epigenetic incidents. These incidents can occur in cells that may vary from endometrial to stem cells. Subtle lesions are viewed as endometrium in a different environment until additional incidents occur. Cystic ovarian or deep endometriosis lesions result from these incidents and are heterogeneous in origin. Simple endometriosis, cystic ovarian endometriosis, and deep endometriosis represent three different diseases that require individualized management.

## 14.5 Hormonal Mechanisms Implicated in Endometriosis

Endometriosis is considered as an estrogen-dependent disorder. This is supported by endometriosis being almost exclusively present in the reproductive period. Earlier work concentrated mostly on the role of estrogen. Later it was realized that the interaction between estrogen and progesterone was just as important. This is not surprising when considering the physiology of endometrial regulation in the reproductive years by the hypothalamic/pituitary/ovarian axis (HPO). The menstrual cycle begins with the production of gonadotropin-releasing hormone (GnRH) by the hypothalamus, which stimulates follicle-stimulating hormone (FSH) and luteinizing hormone (LH) secretion from the anterior pituitary gland. FSH stimulates ovarian follicular development, and together with LH, stimulates estrogen secretion from the follicles. Estrogen subsequently induces endometrial proliferation. A peak in the estrogen level occurs around the 14th day of the menstrual cycle and triggers an LH surge from the pituitary, which leads to ovulation approximately 12 h later. Following ovulation, the corpus luteum secretes progesterone and the estrogen level begins to decline. Progesterone facilitates the transition of proliferative endometrium to secretory endometrium. Secretory transformation is not only critical to prepare the endometrium for implantation but is an essential protective mechanism against uncontrolled endometrial proliferation. In the absence of fertilization, the corpus luteum stops progesterone production. The reduction in serum progesterone and estrogen triggers the start of menses and shedding of the endometrial lining and serves as the signal to the hypothalamus to start a new cycle.

All estrogens are produced from androgen precursors. Most androgen precursors originate from the ovary and to a lesser extent from the adrenal gland. The process by which androgen precursors are converted into estrogens is called aromatization. This process can be accelerated by the excess presence of aromatase enzymes in conditions such as obesity. Under physiological conditions, more potent estradiol (E2) will be converted to less potent estrone (E1). Estrogen exerts effects in the endometrium via two main classical estrogen receptor (ER) isoforms, ERα and ERβ [6]. The progesterone receptor (PR), is a nuclear receptor that is activated by the steroid hormone progesterone. It has two isoforms, PR-A and PR-B. The transcriptional activity of the PR isoforms is affected by specific transcriptional coregulators and by PR post-translational modifications that affect gene promoter targeting. Although some membrane-bound PR exists, their role is presently unclear [7].

Hyper-estrogenism is the first hormonal mechanism that is implicated in endometriosis. This may be secondary to systemic or local causes. Endometriotic tissue has higher local availability of E2 that may be explained by higher aromatase enzyme expression and impaired conversion of potent E2 to less potent E1 [8]. Lack of progesterone or progesterone resistance leads to loss of the protective secretory transformation role of progesterone in the endometrium, thus favoring the progression of endometriotic tissue [9]. Hormonal manipulation can influence the behavior of endometriotic tissue in several ways.

A reduction of systemic estrogen levels can be attained by GnRH agonists or antagonists.

A reduction of estrogenic effects at local levels can be attained by aromatize inhibitors (AI) or selective estrogen receptor modulators (SERMs). Amplification of the progesterone effect on secretory transformation can be attained by progestogens and selective progesterone receptor modulators (SPRMs). The aim of hormonal therapy should be to reduce the size of ectopic endometrial tissue, ameliorate pain, restore fertility, to have an acceptable benefit to risk ratio, to avoid a generalized hypoestrogenic state with consequences such as vasomotor symptoms and bone loss, be suitable for long-term use and be cost-effective [10].

## 14.6 Drugs Commonly Used in Endometriosis

### 14.6.1 Non-hormonal Drugs

#### 14.6.1.1 Non-steroidal Anti-inflammatory Drugs (NSAIDs)

The pain of endometriosis is mediated by increased levels of inflammatory markers such as cytokines, prostaglandins, and interleukins. It is thus comprehensible why in spite of conclusive evidence regarding effectiveness, NSAIDS are often used as first-line drugs against endometriosis-related pain [11]. NSAIDs have a negative gastro-intestinal side effect profile.

### 14.6.2 Hormonal Drugs

#### 14.6.2.1 Combined Hormonal Contraceptives

The European Society of Human Reproduction and Embryology (ESHRE) recommends consideration of combined hormonal contraceptives for the treatment of endometriosis-associated dyspareunia, dysmenorrhea, and non-menstrual pain [1]. It suppresses ovarian hormone activity and leads to increased decidualization of the endometriotic tissue and thereby inhibits the progression of the disease [12]. General acceptance as the most popular form of contraception, relatively low cost, and ease of administration have made combined hormonal contraceptives a popular choice in the treatment of endometriosis. Concern has been expressed that it is often used empirically without an established diagnosis of endometriosis. This may lead to delayed diagnosis of endometriosis, especially deep infiltrating endometriosis. It is recommended to use combinations containing natural estradiol and not synthetic ethynyl estradiol and progestins with a proven strong suppressive effect on endometrial tissue such as dienogest or nomegestrol acetate (NOMAC).

#### 14.6.2.2 GnRH Agonists

GnRH agonists inhibit the production of estrogen at the central level to bring about a medically induced menopause with resultant regression of endometriotic implants. In spite of initially stimulating the release of pituitary FSH and LH, chronic administration leads to the downregulation of pituitary GnRH receptors that results in suppression of the HPO axis leading to a state of hypoestrogenism, anovulation, and effective pain relief [13]. The downside is the consequences of prolonged hypoestrogenism such as bone loss, vaginal atrophy, and vasomotor symptoms. These can be prevented by add-back therapy, usually a combination of low dose estrogen and progestin. The underlying theory of add-back treatment is that the amount of estrogen necessary to prevent hypoestrogenic symptoms and side effects is less than that which would stimulate endometriosis [14]. GnRH agonists are commonly used as a monthly or 3-monthly injection for a period of up to 1 year. Leuprolide acetate, goserelin and nafarelin are available in most countries.

### 14.6.2.3 Gonadotropin-Releasing Hormone Antagonists (GnRH Antagonists)

This group of drugs works by a direct antagonistic effect on pituitary GnRH receptors. This leads to symptomatic relief and regression of the endometriotic lesions, but without causing the initial flare of FSH and LH as seen with GnRH agonists. This leads to a lower degree of hypoestrogenism and a better side effect profile without compromising efficiency. Elagolix has obtained FDA approval for the alleviation of endometriosis-related pain. Elagolix comes in two dosages; 150 mg daily or 200 mg twice daily per mouth [15]. Relugolix 40 mg once daily orally as a fixed dose with add-back therapy of 1 mg estradiol and norethindrone acetate is presently in a stage 3 clinical trial.

### 14.6.2.4 Selective Estrogen Receptor Modulators (SERM)

Selective estrogen receptor antagonism in endometriotic tissue, without a hypoestrogenic side-effect profile, is an attractive proposition in the treatment of endometriosis. Limited trial data suggests that a selective estrogen receptor modulator could be used for the treatment of pain associated with endometriosis [16]. The tissue-specific complex of the SERM bazedoxifene combined with conjugated equine estrogen seems a logical choice but no trial data exists.

### 14.6.2.5 Progestogens

Progesterone has multiple mechanisms of action that explains the rationale of its use in endometriosis. It induces secretory transformation of the endometrium, inhibits estrogen-induced mitosis, alters estrogen receptors, and inhibits angiogenesis and expression of matrix metalloproteinase needed for the growth of the endometriotic implants. Progesterone resistance has been implicated as a major factor in endometriosis. Progestogen therapy has been advocated as first-line therapy in endometriosis treatment. The group of steroid hormones known as progestogens included the natural progestogen, progesterone; the retroprogesterone dydrogesterone as well as several progesterone derivatives (progestins) such as 17-hydroxyprogesterone derivatives and 19-nortestosterone derivatives [17]. Progestogens all bind to progesterone receptors but differ not only with respect to their potency but also in their specificity. Some progestogens also have agonist and/or antagonist effects on estrogen, androgen, glucocorticoid, and mineralocorticoid receptors.

### Dienogest (DNG)

DNG is a 19-nortestosterone derivative with a high affinity for the PR with additional anti-androgenic activity and an antigonadotropic effect. DNG improves progesterone resistance in endometriotic lesions. [18] Although DNG binds to the progesterone receptor with high specificity and produces a potent progestogenic effect, it causes only moderate suppression of estradiol levels, remaining within the lower end of the normal physiological range. Hypoestrogenic side effects as seen with GnRH agonists are thus avoided. Bone loss though has been reported in the first year of treatment and in younger patients [19].

The recommended dosage is 2 mg daily per os. DNG has been shown to be effective in controlling endometriosis-related pelvic pain such as dysmenorrhea, premenstrual pain, and pain associated with deep infiltrating endometriosis. Two studies in Europe and Japan, respectively, with treatment durations up to 65 weeks demonstrated that DNG has an efficacy, safety, and tolerability profile that is favorable for long-term use [20]. Cessation of therapy is associated with prompt restoration of ovulation and fertility.

### Dydrogesterone

Dydrogesterone is a retroprogesterone and a stereoisomer of progesterone, with an additional double-bond between carbon 6 and 7. It is shaped by light from the same natural source as progesterone. Dydrogesterone binds highly selective to the PR resulting in minimal side effects. It effectively relieves endometriosis-related pain and progression of endometriosis lesions. It is approved for these indications in Russia and the Ukraine. It is given orally in a dose of 10–20 mg daily from day 5 to 25. It does not suppress ovulation and pregnancy is possible and feasible.

### Medroxy Progesterone Acetate (MPA)

Although MPA is available as oral tablets, an injectable depo preparation administered 150 mg intramuscularly every 3 months is most commonly used in the treatment of endometriosis. Depo MPA improves endometriosis by a direct effect on endometriotic lesions as well as by ovulation inhibition. In a 6-months study, depo MPA was equivalent to leuprolide (GnRH agonist) in the improvement of endometriosis-related pain but with a lesser effect on bone loss [21].

### Levonorgestrel Containing Intrauterine System (LNG-IUS)

LNG-IUS releases 20 μg of LNG daily in close proximity to the endometrium over a 5-year period. LNG induces atrophy of the endometrium, and a higher concentration of progesterone in the peritoneal cavity leads to suppression of ectopic endometrium by anti-inflammatory and immunomodulatory functions [22]. LNG-IUS has been shown to alleviate endometriosis-related pain. Similar efficacy was reported when compared to GnRH analogs with a lower incidence of hypoestrogenic side effects.

### Selective Progesterone Receptor Modular (SPRMs)

Theoretically, SPRMs should have a beneficial effect on endometriosis-related pain and lesions. Phase 3 trials with Vilaprisan is on temporary hold due to safety concerns. Ulipristal acetate has not been approved for this indication.

### Etonogestrel Implant

It was reported to be equivalent to depot MPA in efficacy to alleviate endometriosis-associated pain as well in side effect profile [23].

## Danazol

Danazol, a derivative of 17 alpha-ethinyl–testosterone, inhibits the LH surge and decreases ovarian steroidogenesis by direct inhibition of ovarian enzymes. In spite of having proven efficacy in relief of endometriosis-associated pain, clinical utility is restricted by an unacceptable hyperandrogenic side effect profile.

## Aromatase Inhibitors (AIs)

Anastrozole, letrozole, and exemestane are third-generation AIs commonly used in the prevention of recurrence of ER-positive breast cancer. Aromatase enzyme facilitates the conversion of steroid precursors into estrogen and is predominantly present in the ovaries and fatty tissue. Aromatase activity is overexpressed in endometriosis [24]. Aromatase-induced estrogen synthesis leads to stimulation of the endometrial implants and an increase in the inflammatory response. In postmenopausal women, the main source of estrogen is peripheral fat. This makes AIs a modality of choice in postmenopausal endometriosis. As in GnRH agonist treatment, the hypoestrogenic side-effect profile can be prevented with add-back therapy.

## 14.7    Future Drugs

Statins, TNFα blockers, anti-angiogenesis factors, and pentoxifylline are drugs currently under investigation for use in endometriosis. There is presently not enough evidence for use in the treatment of endometriosis.

## 14.8    Postmenopausal Endometriosis

Although endometriosis is an estrogen-dependent condition that theoretically should not pose a problem in the postmenopausal period, it may persist into the postmenopause or be reactivated in the postmenopause. As expected, endometriosis is much less common in the postmenopausal period. Endometriotic implants are generally smaller and less active. The most common presenting symptoms are pelvic pain and dyspareunia. It is often associated with autoimmune conditions such as hypothyroidism, rheumatoid arthritis, or lupus [25].

Laparoscopy with biopsy for histological diagnosis is advised. The risk of malignant transformation is higher in the postmenopause, especially in the presence of ovarian endometriosis. This was originally described in 1925 with an estimated incidence of 1% [26]. Surgical removal of endometriotic implants is the treatment of choice. AI is the medical treatment of choice if appropriate.

Menopausal hormone therapy (MHT) should be considered in all cases of surgically induced early menopause including surgery performed for the treatment of endometriosis. Surgical menopause before the age of 45 induces the same hypoestrogenic consequences (especially vasomotor symptoms) as seen with GnRH agonists. The experience with add-back therapy with GnRH agonists has shown that the low levels of MHT needed to treat the hypoestrogenic consequences are below the level required to reactivate endometriotic lesions. MHT may also be considered in the symptomatic women after natural menopause with a previous history of endometriosis, taking into account the benefit to risk ratio in the individual. In the presence of a uterus, combined estrogen/progestogen MHT should be used to eliminate the risk of inducing endometrial carcinoma. In the absence of a uterus, in any patient without endometriosis, unopposed estrogen-only MHT is recommended based on a lower risk of breast cancer when compared to opposed estrogen/progestogen MHT [27]. Based on the understanding of normal physiology of the endometrium and experience with the effect of unopposed estrogen on the endometrium, it is reasonable to assume that unopposed estrogen therapy may stimulate and cause recurrence of endometriosis or favor malignant transformation and that this can be avoided using combined estrogen/progestogen therapy in women with previous endometriosis [28]. The small increased risk of breast cancer associated with combined MHT should be weighed against the risk of stimulation of endometriotic remnants with estrogen-only therapy. It is recommended that all women in need of MHT with a history of endometriosis should be treated with combined estrogen/progestogen MHT in a continuous combined fashion. In order to minimize the risk of breast cancer, it is recommended to use the lowest effective dose. Natural progesterone and dydrogesterone have been shown to have a lower risk of association with breast cancer compared to other progestins. There is insufficient data to make a judgment on whether there is a difference between oral and transdermal therapy. In the case of early menopause, the duration of therapy should be at least till the average age of natural menopause but there is no predetermined limitation on the duration of therapy. It should be consistent with the treatment goals of the individual and the benefit/risk profile needs to be individually reassessed annually. This is important in view of new data indicating a longer duration of vasomotor symptoms in some women.

## 14.9 Conclusion

The aim of this chapter is to empower the reader with the options of hormonal treatment in endometriosis. Insight into the mechanism of actions, efficacy, and side-effect profile will enable the reader to individualize treatment to the best benefit of the victims of endometriosis.

## References

1. Dunselman GA, Vermeulen N, Becker C, et al. European Society of Human Reproduction and Embryology (ESHRE). Guideline: Management of Women with endometriosis. Hum Reprod. 2014;29(3):400–12.
2. Mahmood TA, Templeton A. Prevalence and genesis of endometriosis. Hum Reprod. 1991;6 (4):544–9.
3. Sampson JA. Peritoneal endometriosis due to the menstrual dissemination of endometrial tissue into the peritoneal cavity. Am J Obstet Gynecol. 1927;14:422–69.

4. Macer ML, Taylor HS. Endometriosis and infertility: a review of the pathogenesis and treatment of endometriosis-associated infertility. Obstet Gynecol Clin N Am. 2012;39(4):535–49.
5. Koninckx PR, Ussia A, Adamyan L, et al. Pathogenesis of endometriosis: the genetic/epigenetic theory. Fertil Steril. 2019;111(2):327–40.
6. Hapangama D, Kamal A, Bulmer J. Estrogen receptor β: the guardian of the endometrium. Hum Reprod Update. 2015;21(2):174–93.
7. Patel B, Elguero S, Thakore S, et al. Role of nuclear progesterone receptor isoforms in uterine pathophysiology. Hum Reprod Update. 2015 Mar;21(2):155–73.
8. Bulun SE, Monsivais D, Kakinuma T, et al. Molecular biology of endometriosis: from aromatase to genomic ab- normalities. Semin Reprod Med. 2015;33:220–4.
9. Al-Sabbagh M, Lam EW, Brosens JJ. Mechanisms of endometrial progester-one resistance. Mol Cell Endocrinol. 2012;358:208–15.
10. Karim A, Shafiee M, Aziz N, et al. Reviewing the role of progesterone therapy in endometriosis. Gynecol Endocrinol. 2018;35(1):1–7.
11. Marjoribanks J, Ayeleke R, Farquhar C, et al. Nonsteroidal anti-inflammatory drugs for dysmenorrhoea. Cochrane Database Syst Rev. 2015;30(7):CD001751.
12. Rafique S, DeCherney A. Medical management of endometriosis. Clin Obstet Gynecol. 2017;60(3):485–96.
13. Prentice A, Deary A, Goldbeck-Wood S, et al. Gonadotrophin-releasing hormone analogues for pain associated with endometriosis. Cochrane Database Syst Rev. 2000;2:CD000346.
14. Hornstein M, Surrey E, Weisberg G, et al. Leuprolide acetate depot and hormonal add-back in endometriosis: a 12-month study. Lupron Add-Back Study Group. Obstet Gynecol. 1998;91 (1):16–24.
15. Surrey E, Taylor H, Giudice L, et al. Long-term outcomes of Elagolix in women with endometriosis: results from two extension studies. Obstet Gynecol. 2018 Jul;132(1):147–60.
16. Harada T, Ohta I, Endo Y, et al. Selective estrogen receptor modulator for pain symptoms with endometriosis: an open-label clinical trial. Yonago Acta Med. 2017;60:227–33.
17. Schindler A, Campagnoli C, Druckmann R, et al. Classification and pharmacology of progestins. Maturitas. 2003;46(Suppl 1):S7–S16.
18. Hayashi A, Tanabe A, Kawabe S, et al. Dienogest increases the progesterone receptor isoform B/A ratio in patients with ovarian endometriosis. J Ovarian Res. 2012;5:31.
19. Ebert A, Dong L, Merz M. Dienogest 2 mg daily in the treatment of adolescents with clinically suspected endometriosis: the Visanne study to assess safety in adolescents. J Pediatr Adolesc Gynecol. 2017;30:560–7.
20. Schindler A. Dienogest in long-term treatment of endometriosis. Int J Women's Health. 2011;3:175–84.
21. Crosignani P, Luciano A, Ray A, et al. Subcutaneous depot medroxyprogesterone acetate versus leuprolide acetate in the treatment of endometriosis-associated pain. Hum Reprod. 2006;21(1):248–56.
22. Vercellini P, Vigano P, Somigliana E. The role of the levonorgestrel-releasing intrauterine device in the management of symptomatic endometriosis. Curr Opin Obstet Gynecol. 2005;17 (4):359–65.
23. Walch K, Unfried G, Huber J, et al. Implanon versus medroxyprogesterone acetate: effects on pain scores in patients with symptomatic endometriosis–a pilot study. Contraception. 2009;79 (1):29–34.
24. Bulun S, Zeitoun K, Takayama K, et al. Molecular basis for treating endometriosis with aromatase inhibitors. Hum Reprod Update. 2000;6(5):413–8.
25. Shah D. Postmenopausal endometriosis: an enigma revisited. J Midlife Health. 2014 Oct;5 (4):163–4.
26. Sampson J. Endometrial carcinoma of the ovary, arising in endometrial tissue in that organ. Arch Surg. 1925;10(1):1–72.
27. De Villiers T, Hall J, Pinkerton J, et al. Revised global consensus statement on menopausal hormone therapy. Climacteric. 2016;19(4):313–5.
28. Barrett-Connor E, Slone S, Greendale G, et al. The postmenopausal estrogen/progestin interventions study: primary outcomes in adherent women. Maturitas. 1997;27(3):261–74.

# Endometriosis and Menopause: Realities and Management

**15**

Lydia Marie-Scemama, Marie Carbonnel, and Jean Marc Ayoubi

## 15.1    Introduction

Endometriosis is an estrogen-dependent disease. It predominantly affects reproductive-age women and becomes less active or regresses with the onset of the menopause. Nevertheless, some data from case series and case reports demonstrate that this pathology is, in fact, increasingly reported even after the decrease of ovarian hormonal secretion. Is it a persistence or a recurrence of a premenopausal disease or a new lesion? Does the malignant risk increase with advancing age? (16). Therefore, clinicians must take this into account in the case of pelvic pain affecting the quality of life (QOL) (dysmenorrhea, dyspareunia, chronic pelvic pain), heavy bleeding, or urinary symptoms at this period. Endometriosis can be considered as an intraperitoneal benign proliferation with a "malignant proliferation" like, which can *metastase* to the ovaries, bowel, and even the lungs. Endometriosis is strongly associated with the increased risk of ovarian cancer; this risk is around 2% or 3%.

## 15.2    Definitions

Menopause may be spontaneous or surgically induced. L. Alio et al. [1] remind us of the negative incidence of successive interventions impairing the ovarian reserve inducing the earlier occurrence of the menopause. Ovarian aging is associated with a fall in hormones, especially estrogens. The menopausal symptoms (hot flushes, vaginal dryness, night sweats) are sometimes responsible for negative changes in quality of life. Endometriosis is an enigmatic disease characterized by the development of functional endometrial tissue outside the uterine cavity [2]. This endometrial tissue tending to invade and to seep into the uterine cavity or even further (bowel,

L. Marie-Scemama (✉) · M. Carbonnel · J. M. Ayoubi
Department of Ob Gyn and Reproductive Medicine, Hôpital Foch-Faculté de Médecine Paris Ouest (UVSQ), Suresnes, France

© International Society of Gynecological Endocrinology 2021
A. R. Genazzani et al. (eds.), *Endometriosis Pathogenesis, Clinical Impact and Management*, ISGE Series, https://doi.org/10.1007/978-3-030-57866-4_15

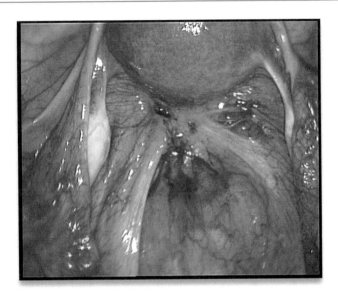

**Fig. 15.1** DIE: Deep infiltrating endometriosis

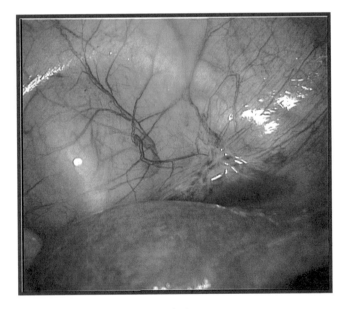

**Fig. 15.2** SUP: Peritoneal superficial endometriosis

ureter, or intrathoracic organs). Endometriosis is a well-known estrogen-dependent disease and heterogeneous in nature with lesions having three distinct phenotypes: superficial peritoneal endometriosis (SUP), ovarian endometrioma (OMA), and deeply infiltrating endometriosis (DIE) (Figs. 15.1, 15.2, and 15.3). Moreover,

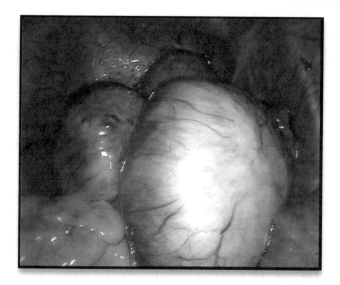

**Fig. 15.3** OMA: Ovarian endometrioma

endometriosis is frequently associated with adenomyosis. The pathogenesis of endometriosis is unclear and it is unknown why different patients present with SUP, OMA, or DIE lesions, and sometimes all the types present in the same patient. The fact that endometriosis phenotype pathogenesis remains unclear suggests that multifactorial mechanisms are involved [3] including hormonal [4], inflammatory [5, 6], immunologic [7, 8], genetic [9–11], epigenetic [12], environmental [13], and other influences. Tan et al. [14] suggest that the endometriotic lesions retained hormonal responsiveness: greater positive progesterone receptor staining and higher positivity of KI-67 antigen [15].

## 15.3 Physiopathology

Data on the physiopathological mechanisms implicated in postmenopausal endometriosis are limited. Around 2–4% of postmenopausal women are estimated to suffer from endometriosis. The fact that endometriosis lesions are able to develop or persist in menopausal women in the absence of menstrual cycles and in a hypo-estrogenic environment sheds doubt on Sampson's physiopathological theory of retrograde bleeding and implicates other mechanisms [16, 17]. During the reproductive years, estrogenic stimulation mainly results from ovarian secretion. At menopause, there is a cessation of menstruation related to a state of ovarian inactivity. However, many issues remain: is it a persistence or a recurrence of a preexisting disease? a de-novo development? a local estrogen production such as found in the case of obesity; phytoestrogens, HRT, or anti-estrogens medications such as Tamoxifen intake? Does stress play a role? What is the relationship with a variant polymorphism

(Genetic-Epigenetic), with hypothyroidism or even the role of fatty acids (unsaturated omega 3)? What is the aromatase role? This was one of the main topics discussed in the last *SEUD (The Society of Endometriosis and Uterine disorders) Conference* (Firenze 2018). Bulun et al. studied estrogen production by endometriosis lesions themselves [17]. According to their work, aromatase is expressed in endometriosis implants and in the ectopic endometrium of women with endometriosis but not in normal endometrium cells; autocrine and paracrine effects result in the local production of estrogens. Estrogens stimulate Cox-2 which increases the formation of prostaglandin E2 and therefore increases aromatase activity. Thus, there is a positive feedback loop in favor of continuous estrogen production in endometriotic lesions. This theory developed by Bulun et al. could explain how endometriosis lesions may persist and become symptomatic in the hypo-estrogenic environment after menopause [18]. This theory is not confirmed by other authors [15]. Certain studies have examined possible sources of estrogens in postmenopausal women that may serve as risk factors for postmenopausal endometriosis. These include obesity, consumption of phytoestrogens, the use of menopausal hormone therapy (MHT), or anti-estrogens such as tamoxifen. There is a possibility that exogenous estrogen will reactivate the growth of endometriotic foci and cause symptomatic recurrence.

## 15.4    Does Endometriosis Persist After Menopause?

Endometriosis is a disease that affects an estimated 6–10% of reproductive-aged women, totaling approximately 176 million women worldwide [17]. Even if endometriosis is more frequent between the years of 25 and 45, it does not disappear after the onset of the menopause. Around 2–4% of postmenopausal women are estimated to suffer from endometriosis [18, 19]. This statement raises three important issues: thinking about the diagnosis, being aware of the role of HRT on recurrence, not forgetting the risk of malignant change with or without HRT, especially in the case of ovarian disease. The case of pain and bleeding should raise our suspicions; Imagery will confirm: Ultrasound and MRI are both necessary. Urinary symptoms as incontinence, more particularly urge incontinence, or dysuria have to be looked for. The first-line treatment for new-onset symptomatic postmenopausal endometriosis should be surgical because of diagnosis uncertainty, the risk of associated malignancy, and the potential risk of subsequent malignant transformation [20]. A laparoscopy will be carried out to fully confirm the diagnosis, to exclude a malignant tumor and, sometimes, to treat the pain surgically. Imaging techniques (transvaginal ultrasound, MRI) are generally not sufficiently accurate to distinguish between endometriosis lesions and cancer. Medical treatment is sometimes prescribed using levonorgestrel IUD, progestin as gestodene or dienogest, or aromatase inhibitors. Levonorgestrel (LNG) IUD is more used in case of adenomyosis; before the menopause, LNG induces a decrease of the endometriosis lesions, especially acting on their size. No post-menopause studies are available. Anti-aromatases as Letrozole; Anastrozole; or Exemestane have been used. They are able to block any extra-ovarian production of estrogens and to induce a decrease of the lesion size and of the pain [21].

## 15.5 Role of HRT

Quality of life of menopausal women is well-known to be affected: changing mood, vaginal dryness, and climacteric syndrome are usually described as feared events by women in this life period. M. Zanello et al. [22] have shown the role of the hypoestrogenic state on bone and cardiovascular disease. Contrary to the 2002 WHI study [23], the new data, published over the last years have shown the interest of using HRT at the beginning of menopause. Hormonal treatment must be started as soon as possible after the menopause. The authors described a "window of opportunity," starting at onset and lasting 10 years. Gemmell [19] and Fedele [24] recently have shown that HRT has a real benefit not only on hot flushes but also on bone health and QOL. It is necessary today, instead of the dissemination of fake news by the WHI, to emphasize the benefit of this treatment over the undefined risks in the case of severely symptomatic women. The benefit on bone and, for many authors, on cardiovascular health has to be taken into consideration, particularly in young patients. The effect of HRT, prescribed at this moment, on the recurrence and malignant transformation risk in women with endometriosis should be considered. In women suffering from severe symptomatic endometriosis undergoing hysterectomy and bilateral salpingo-oophorectomy for pain relief, a combined HRT is usually prescribed, even if their uterus has been removed. If there are resides before the treatment, increased risk exists, especially in the case of significant endometriosis and prescribed to women after menopause in case of significant climacteric symptoms. The authors recommend limited doses of continuous estrogen–progestin. Tibolone is sometimes prescribed [24]. HRT can be given immediately after surgery in the case of bilateral ovariectomy which triggers early menopause. Patients must be informed of the possibility of recurrence. If pain returns, treatment must be stopped. The EMAS statement agrees with these conclusions [25].

## 15.6 Malignant Transformation

Endometriosis is a benign proliferative condition; however, malignant transformation may occur in almost 1% of cases, occurring most commonly in ovarian lesions [26, 27]. Breast cancer and hematopoietic malignancies have been described. Common genetic mutations have been discovered in ovarian cancer and endometriosis (TP53; KRAS; PTEN and mostly ARIDA 14) [28]. In a review, Audebert et al. concluded that endometriosis was strongly associated with the increased risk of ovarian cancer, and Endometriosis Associated Ovarian Cancer (EAOC) showed favorable characteristics including early-stage disease, low-grade disease, and a specific histology such as endometrioid or clear cell carcinoma [29]. In 2016, G. Chene put forward that endometriosis could be a pre-cancerous lesion, which

**Fig. 15.4** Ovarian malignant tumor

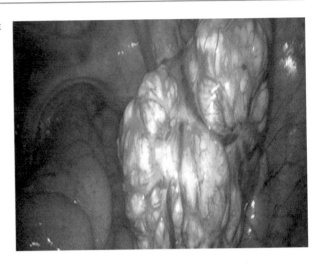

may evolve into atypic hyperplasia and finally into EAOC [30]. Clear cell and endometrioid carcinomas were the malignancies most commonly seen in ovaries containing endometriosis (Fig. 15.4).

## 15.7 Dealing with It

Surgical therapy should be the first-line option for postmenopausal women with symptomatic endometriosis because of the risk of, and the need to exclude, malignancy [31]. If there is a doubt regarding the nature of a postmenopausal pelvic mass, surgery will be proposed to confirm the diagnosis of OMA and to eliminate malignancy or atypia. In the case of pain, it can be used to treat. It is necessary in this case to avoid also the possible complications as utero-hydronephrose or bowel obstruction. Medical therapy may be an option in case of pain recurrence after surgery or if surgery is contraindicated [32]. Levonorgestrel IUD or progestins such as *Gestodene* or Dienogest have been tried out. Also, some data consider using aromatase inhibitors; this kind of medical therapy would block the extra ovarian production of estrogens thus decreasing pain and lesion size [21]. Counselling, yoga, diet, acupuncture, and heating pads can be a real help sometimes, in case of pain.

## 15.8 Conclusion

Postmenopausal endometriosis is a rare condition but a reality which affects 2–4% of women. The origin could be the extra-ovarian production of estrogens by endometriotic lesions and adipose tissue [33]. Endometriotic cells, in this case, would have a tendency to spread and involve extragenital organs, inducing constrictive and obstructive lesions. A multidisciplinary management approach is necessary.

Diagnosis will be carried out through a combination of collecting patient personal history (Pain, Urinary symptoms), conducting a clinical examination and using imagery. In first line, surgical treatment should be used to treat the pain, and to eliminate malignancy. The risk of malignant evolution should not be underestimated: endometrioid, or clear cell carcinoma. In more complex cases, the patient should be referred to a specialized endometriosis unit. Medical therapy should come in second line: aromatase inhibitors, levonorgestrel-IUD, progestins. HRT may increase recurrence risk. Nevertheless, it is imperative, before refusing to prescribe, to weigh up the risks and benefits. Data are insufficient to justify an automatic refusal to prescribe HRT, especially in the case of premature menopause.

# References

1. Alio L, et al. Endometriosis: seeking optimal management in women approaching menopause. Climacteric. 2019;22(4):329–38.
2. Sampson JA. Metastatic or embolic endometriosis due to premenstrual dissemination of endometrial tissue into the peritoneal cavity. Am J Obstet Gynecol. 1927;3:93–110.
3. Vercellini P, Vigano P, Somigliana E, Fedele L. Endometriosis: pathogenesis and treatment. Nat Rev Endocrinol. 2014;10:261–75.
4. Burney RO, Talbi S, Hamilton AE, Vo KC, Nezhat CR, Lessey BA, Giudice LC. Gene expression analysis of endometrium reveals progesterone resistance and candidate susceptibility genes in women with endometriosis. Endocrinology. 2007;148:3814–26.
5. Santulli P, Borghese B, Noel JC, Fayt I, Anaf V, de Ziegler D, Batteux F, Vaiman D, Chapron C. Hormonotherapy deregulates prostaglandin-endoperoxidase synthase (PTGS2) expression in endometriotic tissues. J Clin Endocrinol Metab. 2014;99:881–90.
6. Santulli P, Chouzenoux S, Fiorese M, Marcellin L, Lemarechal H, Millischer AE, Batteux F, Borderie D, Chapron C. Protein oxidative stress markers in peritoneal fluids of women with deep infiltrating endometriosis are increased. Hum Reprod. 2015;30:49–60.
7. Leconte M, Nicco C, Ngo C, Chereau C, Chouzenoux S, Marut W, Guibourdenche J, Arkwright S, Weill B, Chapron C, Dousset B, Batteux F. The mTOR/AKT inhibitor temsirolimus prevents deep infiltrating endometriosis in mice. Am J Pathol. 2011;179:880–9.
8. Ngo C, Nicco C, Leconte M, Chereau C, Arkwright S, VAcher Lavenu MC, Weill B, Chapron C, Batteux F. Protein kinase inhibitors can control the progression of endometriosis in vitro and in vivo. J Pathol. 2010;222:148–57.
9. Borghese B, Tost J, de Surville M, Busato F, Letourneur F, Mondon F, Vaiman D, Chapron C. Identification of susceptibility genes for peritoneal, ovarian, and deep infiltrating endometriosis using a pool sample-based genome-wide association study. Biomed Res Int. 2015;2015:461024.
10. Nyholt DR, et al. Genome-wide association meta-analysis identifies new endometriosis risk loci. Nat Genet. 2012;44:1355–9.
11. Pagliardini L, Gentilini D, Vigano P, Panina-Bordignon P, Busacca M, Candiani M, Di Blasio AM. An Italian association study and meta-analysis with previous GWAS confirm WNT4, CDKN2BAS and FN1 as the first identified susceptibility loci for endometriosis. J Med Genet. 2013;50:43–6.
12. Borghese B, Barbaux S, Mondon F, Santulli P, Pierre G, Vinci G, Chapron C, Vaiman D. Research resource: genome wide profiling of methylated promoters in endometriosis. Mol Endocrinol. 2010;24:1872–8.
13. Umezawa M, Sakata C, Tanaka N, Tabata M, Takeda K, Ihara T, Sugamata M. Pathological study for the effects of in utero and postnatal exposure to diesel exhaust on a rat endometriosis model. J Toxicol Sci. 2011;36:493–8.

14. Tan DA, Almaria MJ. Postmenopausal endometriosis: drawing a clearer clinical picture. Climateric. 2018;21(3):249–55.
15. Toki T, et al. Proliferative activity of postmenopausal endometriosis: a histopathologic and immunocytochemical study. Int J Gynecol Pathol. 1996;15(1):45–53.
16. Bendon CL, Becker CM. Potential mechanisms of postmenopausal endometriosis. Maturitas. 2012;72:214–9.
17. Bulun SE. Endometriosis. N Engl J Med. 2009;360:268–79.
18. Bulun SE, Yang S, Fang Z, Gurates B, Tamura M, Sebastian S. Estrogen production and metabolism in endometriosis. Ann N Y Acad Sci. 2002;955:396–40.
19. Gemmell LC, Webster KE, Kirtley S, Vincent K, Zondervan KT, Becker CM. The management of menopause in women with a history of endometriosis: a systematic review. Hum Reprod Update. 2017;23(4):481–500.
20. Soliman NF, Hillard TC. Hormone replacement herapy in women with past history of endometriosis. Climateric. 2006;9:325–35.
21. Polyzos NP, Fatemi HM, Zavos A, Papanikolau EG. Aromatase inhibitors in post menopausal endometriosis. Reprod Biol Endocrinol. 2011;9:90.
22. Zanello M, et al. Hormonal replacement therapy in menopausal women with history of endometriosis: a review of literature. Medicina (Kaunas). 2019;55(8):477.
23. Writing Group for the Women's Health Initiative Investigator. Risks and benefits of estrogen plus progestin in healthy postmenopausal women. Principal results from the women's health initiative randomized controlled trial. JAMA. 2002;288:321–33.
24. Fedele L, Bianchi S, Raffaelli R, Zanconato G. Comparison of transdermal estradiol and tibolone for the treatment of oophorectomized women with deep residual endometriosis. Fertil Steril. 1989;51(5):781–5.
25. EMAS Position Statement: Managing the Menopause in Women with a Past History of Endometriosis. Moen MH. European menopause and Andropause society. Maturitas. 2010;67 (1):94–7.
26. Stern RC, Dash R, Bentley RC, Snyder MJ, Haney AF, Robboy SJ. Malignancy in endometriosis: frequency and comparison of ovarian and extraovarian types. Int J Gynecol Pathol. 2001;20:133–9.
27. Melin A, SParen P, Perrson I, Bergqvist A. Endometriosis and the risk of cancer with special emphasis on ovarian cancer. Hum Reprod. 2006;21:1237–42.
28. Wiegand KC, et al. ARID1A mutations in endometriosis-associated ovarian carcinomas. N Engl J Med. 2010;363(16):1532–43.
29. Audebert A. Women with endometriosis: are they different from others? Gynecol Obstet Fertil. 2005;33(4):239–46.
30. Chene G. L'endométriose est elle une lesion pré cancéreuse? Perspectives et implications cliniques. Gynécol Obstét Fertil. 2016;44:106–12.
31. Inceboz U. ENdometriosis after menopause. Womens Health (Lond). 2015;11:711–5.
32. Streuli I, Gaitzch H, Wenger JM, Petignat P. Endometriosis after menopause: physiopathology and management of an uncommon condition. Climateric. 2017;20:138–43.
33. Chapron C, Marcellin L, Borghese B, Santulli P. Rethinking mechanisms, diagnosis and management of endometriosis. Nat Rev Endocrinol. 2019;15:666–82.

Printed in the United States
by Baker & Taylor Publisher Services